the Metabolism Plan

Discover the Foods and Exercises That
Work for Your Body to Reduce
Inflammation and Lose Weight Fast

LYN-GENET RECITAS

Every effort has been made to ensure that the information in the book is accurate. The information in this book may not be applicable in each individual case so it is advised that professional medical advice is obtained for specific health matters and before changing any medication or dosage. Neither the publisher nor author accepts any legal responsibility for any personal injury or other damage or loss arising from the use of the information in this book. The advice herein is not intended to replace the services of trained health professionals, or be a substitute for medical advice. In addition if you are concerned about your diet or exercise regime and wish to change them, you should consult a health practitioner first.

First published in 2017 by Grand Central Life & Style
An imprint of Grand Central Publishing

This edition first published in Great Britain in 2017
by Orion
an imprint of The Orion Publishing Group Ltd
Carmelite House, 50 Victoria Embankment
London EC4Y 0DZ

An Hachette UK Company

1 3 5 7 9 10 8 6 4 2

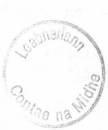

A CIP catalogue record for this book
is available from the British Library.

ISBN: 978 1 4091 6236 0

Printed in Great Britain by CPI Group (UK) Ltd, Croydon, CR0 4YY

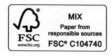

www.orionbooks.co.uk

This book, a true labor of love, is dedicated to my family first. Thank you, Bill, for your love and patience. To my incredible son Brayden, you light up my life and are God's blessing to me. To Ella, you are a testament to what a healing diet can accomplish. Ted Recitas, thanks for always being part of the family and having our back. Lastly, to my Metabolism Planners, every day you inspire me and teach me more about courage and the incredible drive to always feel your best. I couldn't have written this book without your hard work!

Contents

Part Three

YOUR METABOLISM PLAN FOR LIFE   235

A Health Plan Just for You

"I've been on half a dozen diets and followed every one to the letter. I lose weight for the first week, but then it all piles back on and I gain back even more, even though I practically live at the gym!"

"I've tried every diet there is—vegan, Paleo, you name it. Now I'm on a no-carbs, no-sugar, and no-fruit diet. They all work for a little while—but then I gain back even more than I lost. At this point maybe I should be on the no-food diet!"

"If I basically starve myself and exercise to death, I can lose weight—but the moment I start to have a life, it all comes back on."

Does this sound like you? Smart, motivated, disciplined—and totally unsuccessful when it comes to losing weight and keeping it off?

Well, I've got some great news for you: It's not your fault. You've been told to count calories, focus on "healthy" foods, and exercise until it hurts—right? But guess what: That advice is completely wrong. Instead, if you want to lose weight you need to:

1. Stop counting calories.
2. Stop eating healthy foods.
3. Stop exercising so darn much.

Does that sound completely counterintuitive? I've been helping people use The Plan precepts to lose weight for more than a decade, and I promise you—it's true. As a nutritionist, yoga instructor, and best-selling author who has worked with tens of thousands of clients, I have seen what works and what doesn't. What I'm going to tell you in this book works. What you've been doing before you got here probably doesn't.

Calorie counting doesn't work. Plain and simple. If it did, we would all be skinny. There would be no way we could gain 3 pounds in one day. If calorie counting worked, you wouldn't be beating yourself up right now for your body not "responding."

Healthy foods? There is no such thing—only what is healthy *for you*. Each of us is chemically unique, which means that a food that works for me might trigger a weight-gaining sensitivity in you. Your weight—and your health in general—is basically your chemical response to food. This little scientific truth is very good news indeed, because it means that when you find the foods that work for you, you will have optimal weight and health. For example, I gain an entire pound every time I have one little 70-calorie egg, while eggs may be the healthiest food for you. We're all different—and calories have nothing to do with that.

And then there's exercise, which has become the new diet religion, the thing that's supposed to be good for everybody all the time, and the more, the better. But here's the truth: If you exercise too intensely for your body, you'll gain weight because you'll drive up your levels of inflammation and *cortisol*, a stress hormone that can slow your metabolism and cause you to gain weight. Cortisol plus inflammation can wreak total havoc in your body, causing weight gain, hormonal and metabolic issues, and even illness.

How can all the diet information you've been hearing about for years be so wrong? Well, the health information you've been getting—whether from diet books, websites, or your favorite health guru—is based on what works for "most people," "average" responses that are true for the "general population." But you are *not* average! You are unique and complex, and you deserve to know what works specifically for *you*, which might very well be completely different from what works for "most people."

The diet gurus try to hedge their bets by putting as many foods as possible on the "forbidden" list. Anything that might be a problem for *someone* gets taken off the table for *everyone*—including you. No fats, no gluten, no sugar, no dairy...it seems like every day, another list of foods gets demonized. Page after page of weight-loss advice steers you away from "danger foods," with involved scientific explanations for why they cause you to gain weight. Just as many pages steer you toward supposedly healthy choices: salmon, turkey, egg whites, spinach, cauliflower, and yogurt. In theory, you can lose weight on these foods. But what if you can't? What if the experts are looking at the problem in the wrong way?

With all these impossible rules, your body starts to feel like the enemy. So you tie yourself up in knots, asking the waiter for tomatoes instead of toast, and steaming up cauliflower instead of baking a potato. Yet you can't lose weight, and you're miserable. Eating has stopped being satisfying, let alone enjoyable, because every choice is a constant battle in a war you can never really win.

If that's true for food, it goes double for exercise. The experts agree: Exercise is good for you, and the more, the better. So you drag yourself out of bed each morning to get in that hour on the treadmill or trudge over to the gym after work to lift weights. No matter how hard you work out, how many extra sessions you book at the gym, your body just isn't responding in the ways the experts say it should.

Or maybe you've got the opposite problem. Maybe believing that you need to exercise at least five hours a week has kept you from exercising at all. Maybe you could manage a few minutes a day, a few days a week, but the experts have you thinking, "What's the point?" so you don't even begin.

What's the solution?

Learn what works for *you*. I've been working for more than 25 years as a nutritionist, and my book *The Plan* not only is a *New York Times* bestseller but has been published in more than 15 countries. It has shown hundreds of thousands of people how to find the foods that are right *for them* so they can lose weight, feel great, and regain their health. My work is in line with all the latest research: Study after study now acknowledges that *bio-individuality*—an individualized diet that works for your personal chemistry—is the only effective way to lose weight and keep it off forever.

My first book, *The Plan*, gave readers the tools to do just that, using a program I developed and have perfected over the years with clients at my health center in New York City. In this book, I take my original Plan to the next level. *The Metabolism Plan* will show you exactly how eating the right foods *for you* supports your metabolism, while eating the wrong foods *for you* sabotages your metabolism. Bio-individuality is the weight-loss secret that no one has told you about—until now.

In this book, you'll also learn why your thyroid is the key to weight loss, energy, and overall well-being, and how you can rev up your metabolism by supporting your thyroid. You'll even find out that sleeping more can be one of your most powerful weight-loss tools—seriously! Last but definitely not least, you'll learn a bio-individual approach to exercise, finding out which types of exercise and lifestyle choices work for your body, and which sap your metabolism and create weight gain.

I'm thrilled with *The Metabolism Plan* because this book represents the latest and most successful stage in my work with clients, expanding on my success with *The Plan*. In that book, I shared one key piece of the puzzle: the importance of choosing the foods that are right *for you*— foods that work for *your* biochemistry. Since that book was published, I've realized that there is another crucial piece that can make weight loss even more effective: your *metabolism*. Yes, choosing the right foods is absolutely vital—but so is supporting metabolic function by taking care of your thyroid, choosing the exercise that's right for your body, and getting the sleep and stress relief your metabolism needs to function at its best. *The Plan* gave you the basics: how to choose the foods that support your own unique body chemistry. But when I saw people gaining weight from doing too much exercise, when I saw how stress and insufficient sleep were disrupting metabolism and sabotaging weight loss, I knew I had to write this book to give you the rest of the story. You're working too hard not to have the best results.

Your body can seem like an impossibly complicated puzzle. But once you have the right information, that puzzle becomes remarkably easy to solve. So stop worrying, my good friend. Relax, the weight-loss and fitness solution you've been looking for all your life has finally arrived. And you know why it works? Because it's all about you.

Jenny, Age 46

Prior to discovering *The Metabolism Plan* I struggled with weight loss—and I mean struggled. I tried all the diets and different ways of eating. I exercised like crazy! I ran a marathon and didn't even lose a pound while training. Not a pound! I did p90X workouts and took spinning classes...none of it helped with weight loss.

Then I found *The Plan* and it made perfect sense, so I began working with Lyn-Genet. Weight loss from diet alone was still slow, so Lyn suggested we add some exercise. After I reigned in my "don't dare ask me to exercise because that doesn't work for me!" attitude, I began to listen to what she had to say. Just to appease Lyn, I started with 7 to 8 minutes every second day. Much to my skeptical eye the weight loss increased. I was wowed! We slowly, and I mean *slowly*, increased the time I spent exercising, but I've never spent more than 30 minutes working out since I started. I now relish in the fact that I've lost almost 50 pounds—*without* long workouts. I am so thankful for finding this approach to food and exercise! I'm in my 40s and have never looked or felt better! Thanks, Lyn-Genet!

Stress Is Slowing Your Metabolism and Making You Sick

It is *not* your imagination. Yes, you are gaining weight and you can blame stress for your expanding waistline. But the effects of stress don't end there. Feel like you're running on fumes? That's stress. Depressed, raging hormones, snapping at coworkers and your kids? That's stress, too. And, worse, premature aging and chronic illness are all by-products of the S word. A never-ending list of to-do's, job pressures, family stressors, exercising too intensely, and constant exposure to technology are some of the reasons why we feel like there's never enough time and that we are ten steps behind.

Why does stress affect us so much? And, more important, what can we do about it? Stress, in and of itself, is not necessarily bad. In fact, we need the stress response to fight infections and keep us safe. A stress response can also mean excitement—think of a first date or the thrill of a job promotion. The issue with stress is when it doesn't go away and becomes chronic. When the periods of stress are too high and you don't have enough of a relaxation response, your body goes haywire.

In my practice, I always look at thyroid hormones and two hormones I like to call your "base hormones": DHEA and pregnenolone. Low levels of DHEA and pregnenolone are signs that your adrenal system is under great stress. Pregnenolone is produced in our adrenals and is the base hormone from which nearly all other steroid hormones are made, including cortisol, DHEA, progesterone, testosterone, and estrogen. When someone deals with chronic stress on a regular basis, more of the pregnenolone is used to feed production of cortisol. As cortisol levels rise, it reduces the production of DHEA, which is known as the fountain of youth. Okay, now this is starting to sound bad, right? DHEA is used to make all your sex hormones, like estrogen and testosterone, and it is critical for fat-burning and lean muscle mass, as well as immune system balance.

Ideally, when the stress is gone, pregnenolone, cortisol, and DHEA levels should go back to normal. However, when the stress is prolonged and occurs for too long, sometimes the body does not recover or bring these hormones back to normal levels even when stress is lessened. Instead, your body remains in crisis mode with high cortisol and low DHEA output. If this continues for long enough, your body will get to the point where even cortisol levels will drop because your other hormones have become so depleted. This is known as adrenal burnout.

Adrenal dysfunction can also cause autoimmune issues to flare up because stress weakens and disrupts digestion. The most common side effect of chronic stress is the development of a leaky gut–type syndrome, where large proteins and antigens pass through the intestinal barrier. These proteins and antigens trigger an immune response and are strongly implicated in triggering autoimmune disorders as a result. This also means that the food sensitivities you have will heighten and you will start to put on more weight in reaction to these reactive foods. More and more foods become inflammatory over time, which results in an inability to lose weight. This syndrome also causes digestive disorders like IBS, chronic constipation, and Crohn's disease. These effects on digestion all heighten the levels of chronic inflammation, which also means premature aging and heightened risk for diseases like type 2 diabetes, heart disease, and even cancer.

Adrenal stress and the inflammation it causes can also lead to thyroid hormone resistance by making your cells less able to "accept" the thyroid hormone's stimulation. This means that, even if your thyroid numbers read in a "normal range" and even if you're taking thyroid medications, your body may be resistant to the thyroid stimulation that is essential for optimal metabolism, mood sex drive, and energy levels. Since the thyroid is essential for every metabolic and cellular function, this will further worsen weight gain.

How do you know if you are having adrenal issues? Simple blood work can help you determine your stress levels and we can put you on a regimen to restore you back to optimal weight, health, and mood. Ask your doctor to test your hormones and include DHEA and pregnenolone as part of your blood work.

How I Developed The Metabolism Plan

I want to share with you the story of how I developed The Plan, which has since evolved into The Metabolism Plan. I suffered terribly from near-daily migraines from the time I was five and went to doctor after doctor trying to find answers. Nothing helped, and the drugs they gave me only numbed the pain without making me feel really well. I refused to believe that there was nothing more to be done, so I kept reading health books trying to find an answer to my near-constant pain. I even started practicing yoga at the age of 11.

When I was 14, I had found my answer: I became a vegetarian. I had discovered a whole new world, one where I felt great every day. I also realized that I loved to cook, and I started baking in health food restaurants that very year!

That was how I began what would turn out to be a lifetime practice: solving my problems through changing what I ate and how I exercised. Today, I would say, "I found the foods and movement that my body loved, and avoided the foods and exercise that weren't right for my particular chemistry." At 14, all I knew was that once I gave up certain foods and practiced yoga, my whole life changed. I went from being a low-energy, slightly depressed teen to becoming a vital, optimistic person who was pretty much always at "110 percent." It was my first lesson in the power of food and exercise—and it was a powerful lesson.

Over the years, I studied holistic nutrition, homeopathy, herbology, and Eastern medicine. I started practicing as a nutritionist, kept working in the hottest restaurants, and even became a sommelier! Good food and excellent wine have always been an integral part of my life, and I want them to be part of yours, too. Eventually, though, working in restaurants just wasn't offering me enough fulfillment. So in 2000, I decided to devote myself full-time to wellness.

Since then I've owned and directed a yoga studio, run a physical therapy center, and opened a holistic health center. I also shared with my clients the three-day food-based cleanse I had been using myself—a cleanse that has brought us all remarkable results for more than 25 years. During the cleanse, my clients stuck to a few select foods, primarily fresh vegetables, fruit, and seeds, all chosen to provide optimal nutrition. The people who went on the cleanse felt great, got rid of symptoms, and generally lost 5 pounds or more.

After the cleanse, I gave my clients a list of healthy foods—and that's when some of them started having trouble. Although they had easily lost weight during the cleanse, many people inexplicably gained 1 or 2 pounds in a single day—even though they were still eating only foods that I had been taught were super healthy.

One person would gain weight with beans, another with salmon, yet another with yogurt or strawberries. What was going on?

It wasn't only weight gain. Immediately after eating a supposedly "healthy" food, many people began to feel unwell. Headaches, indigestion, constipation, aching joints, depression—my patients responded within minutes and almost violently to the foods that were supposed to be good for them.

This was when I first realized that different people had vastly different responses to foods—even foods that were supposed to be healthy. I also understood that their intensely negative responses were partly because the cleanse had done such a good job of allowing their bodies to heal. Once freed of all the unhealthy foods that had been weighing them down, their bodies were quick to reject any other foods that didn't really work. Symptoms that are muffled and "under the radar" when your body has gotten used to a problematic food suddenly emerge dramatically when you have cleansed your body of that food. If you eat even a little of a food that doesn't work for you, your body says *loud* and *clear,* "Please don't feed this to me!"

Certain patterns of seemingly "perfect" started to emerge. Keeping careful records, I discovered that 85 percent of my clients had negative reactions—weight gain, symptoms, emotional issues—when they consumed salmon, asparagus, Greek yogurt, or strawberries. And 70 percent had negative reactions to walnuts, green peppers, and tofu. Another group of foods provoked negative reactions in 60 percent, 50 percent, 40 percent, and so on. I kept tracking people's responses until I ultimately came up with the reactive food chart you can see on page 14.

The more data I collected, the more astounded I was: Seemingly "healthy" foods were the exact opposite of health promoting for many people—and everyone's reaction was different. But what was the problem with these foods? Why were they provoking all these symptoms?

The answer is inflammation, an immune-system response to any type of injury or infection that your body considers a threat. Inflammation is meant to help your body rid itself of bacteria or viruses that threaten your health, and to help your body repair injured or infected tissue.

However, this healing response can also produce troublesome effects, including weight gain and a wide range of symptoms. (You'll learn more about this in Chapter 1, starting on page 3.) Apparently, certain foods were triggering inflammation in my clients, resulting in weight gain and a whole host of physical, mental, and emotional symptoms.

I had already been researching the effects of inflammation, so I was able to see how well it applied to the results I had noticed in my clients. I had learned that *chronic* inflammation—inflammation that never really goes away—is behind many of the diseases of our time: cardiovascular disease, diabetes, autoimmune disorders, and cancer. As I realized how many foods caused inflammation, I was intrigued and thrilled by a new idea. Maybe we could address these chronic illnesses by lowering inflammation—which we could do by changing people's diets. It wouldn't work simply to tell people, "Don't eat unhealthy foods." What we'd have to do is figure out which foods were unhealthy *for them*—which foods triggered inflammation in their own particular chemistry. *Those* were the foods they would have to avoid. *Those* were the foods—the only foods—that were causing them to feel sick and to gain weight.

The key was how different each person's chemistry can be—how each one of us reacts to different triggers. That's why some of my clients couldn't tolerate salmon while others reacted badly to yogurt—each unique immune system was having its own specific reaction. I also realized that inflammation produces a different cluster of symptoms in each of us: One client might develop headaches in response to a trigger food, while another got indigestion and a third responded with anxiety. We might even develop different symptoms at different times in our lives: constipation in our 20s; aching joints and irritable bowel syndrome (IBS) in our 30s; Crohn's disease, depression, and hormonal issues in our 40s. Still, the underlying cause of all these problems is the same: *inflammation*, the response of an alarmed immune system.

When I was making these discoveries, the prevailing theory was that obesity caused inflammation—but I was seeing something very different. It seemed that weight gain was also *caused* by inflammation—that is, by the inflammatory reaction that people have when they eat a food that triggers a negative response. That negative response always included both physiological symptoms and weight gain. Light bulb moment: Healthy foods could cause inflammation.

I continued to gather data from my clients, tracking their diets and their symptoms. I had people email me daily—even hourly!—a practice that my staff and I still use today. This stream of real-time data allowed me to monitor exactly how food choices affected my clients' weight, health, and mood. A couple of hundred case studies later, I had the basics of a new approach to eating, which I called The Plan. That became the basis for a *New York Times* bestseller.

Since publishing *The Plan*, I've continued to hone my approach, learning where it worked and where I could make it more effective. For most people, *The Plan* worked beautifully, but some of my clients were noticing they gained weight on days when they should have lost. As I began exploring this in depth, I realized that diet was just one piece of the body's very complex puzzle. True healing and reliable, consistent, long-term weight loss couldn't really begin until I factored exercise into the equation and until I'd addressed any underlying issues with the thyroid: the magic key to weight loss, energy, and overall wellness. Eventually I developed a new program: The Metabolism Plan.

This new program shares with the old one a radical new approach to eating and exercise, based on decades of research, development, and in-the-trenches experience. But thanks to the new data I gathered and the new insights I developed, The Metabolism Plan works even better than its predecessor, and I'm thrilled to share it with you.

I'm also excited that, like The Plan, The Metabolism Plan allows you to enjoy many of your favorite foods, to quickly and steadily lose weight, and to feel healthier and more energized than ever before. Even better, after a few months on The Metabolism Plan, your digestion will improve as inflammation subsides. This will allow you to tolerate many foods you may have had to cut out of your diet. I can't tell you the look of joy on people's faces as they are able to bring back in wheat or dairy after years of avoiding these foods!

What if I've Already Read *The Plan*?

I'm so happy you have read *The Plan*! You're going to love reading this book, too, and you can think of yourself as an advanced student!

What you learned in *The Plan*—and what you will find here as well—is a master class in choosing the foods that are right for your body while avoiding the foods your body doesn't do well with. But in *The Metabolism Plan*, you'll go much deeper into figuring out your chemistry, because this book does for exercise what *The Plan* did for food: It teaches you exactly which types of exercise work for your body and which types don't. Learning how to test exercise, just as you know how to test food, is going to be crucial for boosting your metabolism.

You will also get an in-depth explanation of all the other factors that affect your metabolism: thyroid health, sleep, and stress. Once you understand what your body needs in all these areas, your weight will be even easier to maintain, and your symptoms will truly disappear, once and for all. Get ready to say goodbye to fatigue, anxiety, depression, joint pain, headaches, digestive issues, and problems with your hormones. Get ready to feel "110 percent" every moment of your life.

Sounds good, yes? Here's a bonus: You'll also find an exciting new Plan designed for even better weight loss and healing.

Deanna, Age 47

I am a 47-year-old woman who at the age of 40 hit a wall and gradually gained weight until my "always 125 pounds" body weighed 165. I would repeatedly go on a diet, lose a few pounds, and then in a flash go right back to my high weight. I couldn't understand it, because I was "eating clean." I eliminated bread, butter, baked goods—my motto was, "If it tastes decadent, spit it out." It came to the point where I was limiting myself to 1,200 calories a day—and still the scale did not budge!

On New Year's Day I ran into an old friend who told me his sister had lost 40 pounds by working with Lyn-Genet. I laughed and said, "How much is it going to cost me?" I was shocked to hear I only had to buy healthy food, plus a few supplements if my body needed them. The immediate 5-pound loss during the cleanse was serious motivation to keep going.

My *aha* moment came on the day I was able to test a new break-fast choice. I went with my former go-to health breakfast: fresh yogurt from the farmer's market. The next morning I weighed 2 whole pounds more than the day before! I learned my lesson and pulled all cow's dairy out of my diet. I'm no longer dragging in the afternoons, the acne I have struggled with since I was 12 years old is nonexistent, and I no longer have symptoms of perimenopause.

This way of eating has given me a quality of life I didn't know was still available to me. I never thought bread, butter, baked goods, and chocolate would be part of my life again. I'm doing things I never imagined I would: exercising, cooking, drinking red wine, even buy-ing vegan cheese—the biggest shock of all to those who know me. The most exciting part of all of this is that I now know with The Metabolism Plan I can be healthy for the rest of my life.

PS. It's a lot of fun getting rid of my fat clothing!

Diet and Exercise: What Most People Are Doing Wrong

I work all day, every day with people like you who are trying to lose weight and get healthier. I'm always hearing about what people think is the right approach to weight loss—what they've heard from their doctor or nutritionist, what they've read in the latest magazine, what worked for their best friend. I've got to tell you, it makes me want to cry, because almost every time, the advice that they are killing them-selves to follow is just plain wrong.

I can boil down their mistakes to one sentence: Instead of creating their own personal plan, geared to their own unique biochemistry, they followed the general advice that's supposed to work for "most people."

Now, if that general advice works for you, great. But if it doesn't—if the only way you can lose weight is by virtually starving yourself or spending every spare hour at the gym, and especially if even that doesn't work—then listen up. Because here is the true secret to weight loss:

Stop following general recommendations based on what is "normal" or "typical"—the foods that may be healthy or unhealthy for "most people."
Instead, develop a personalized plan specifically tailored to your own unique body chemistry.

Once you learn how to create your own personalized plan, you can rely on this method for the rest of your life. Whether you're in your 20s, 80s, or anywhere in between, creating a personalized plan will work for you—and it will keep on working. The beauty of The Metabolism Plan is that you always have the tools to figure out exactly what your body needs.

I always say you've got two choices:

1. You can spend 40 or 50 or even 60 years dieting...
2. or you can invest 30 days in figuring out your own chemistry and never have to count a calorie again.

This is the book that's going to teach you how to create that wonderful new life. First, you'll find that your excess weight comes off quickly and easily. You consume at least 2,000 calories a day, you never feel hungry, and you're eating delicious meals and snacks that might well include foods that have been off-limits to you for years: guacamole, cheese, wine, chocolate. At the end of your first 30 days on The Metabolism Plan, you'll have a customized weight-loss program and all the know-how you need to continue to lose weight (if you desire) or to maintain your healthy new weight.

What will you discover in those 30 days? Will you have to lose some of your favorite foods? Not necessarily! In fact, you might even find that foods you thought you had to give up—French fries, bread, rice—work great for your chemistry, promoting optimal weight loss and health. It may be that some foods do cause weight gain—but you don't have to say goodbye to these foods forever. When your metabolism is operating at peak condition, you can indulge in thin-crust pizza, cake, or fried calamari. Even if you do gain weight from eating a food, a little gain is fine, because all you have to do is go back to the foods that work for you and you can lose weight any day you want to! It's only when you have inflammatory day after inflammatory day that you get sick and have trouble staying at a healthy weight.

You'll get even better results because on The Metabolism Plan, you are supporting your own specific food plan with your own personalized exercise plan. News flash: Most people are exercising incorrectly. If you've been working out more than 20 minutes a day, three days a week, you might be stressing your body and making it harder to lose weight. You might also be doing the wrong type of exercise for your body. In this book, I'll teach you how to exercise based on your body's natural energy levels. That's the key to more weight loss and improved metabolism.

You deserve your own plan, geared to your own unique body. I don't want you slogging away for a self-defeating hour on the elliptical. I want you doing the smart exercises that your body loves! In Chapter 5, I show you how to create that personal plan, with exactly the type and amount of exercise that is right for you.

The Thyroid Factor

A fully functioning thyroid means your metabolism is operating at full blast, which is what you want for optimal weight loss. In this book, you'll learn all the factors that can affect your thyroid's function—diet, exercise, sleep, and stress—so you can keep your thyroid happy.

That's important, because when your thyroid is happy, you're happy. Good thyroid function means you lose excess weight without even trying. You feel totally energized. Your mind is clear and sharp, your mood is calm and optimistic, and your skin and hair look great.

Sounds good, right? But when your thyroid is dysfunctional, you feel you have hit rock bottom, and you're in a constant struggle with your body. You gain weight at the drop of a hat. You feel sluggish and foggy, and you frequently struggle with mood swings, hair loss, low sex drive, or digestive issues.

So in this book, I'll show you exactly how to keep your thyroid in peak shape and teach you how to measure thyroid function using the simplest of tools: an over-the-counter thermometer. I want you to take charge of your own metabolism—and when you've mastered The Metabolism Plan, you can!

Stress and Sleep

Nothing saddens me more than when people keep dragging themselves through the day on five or six hours of sleep—and then wonder why they can't lose weight. Here's the deal: If your body isn't getting the sleep it needs, your thyroid can't function properly and your metabolism goes awry. Now you're gaining weight, even when you stick faithfully to a Spartan diet. It really is that simple, which is why you need to make sure that you get the amount of sleep that is right for you.

Another thing I hear all the time is how stressed my clients are. When I ask what they are doing for stress relief, they look at me blankly. "I thought we were here to talk about weight loss," many of them say.

"We are!" I answer. Stress causes weight gain. It can majorly disrupt your body chemistry, packing on the pounds faster than a double serving of chocolate cake. Don't worry, because I'll show you how to relieve your stress, soothe your body chemistry, and get your metabolism back on track.

A Health Plan Just for You

Whether we're talking about diet, exercise, stress, or sleep, it all comes down to the same thing: developing a personalized Plan that is perfect for your own personal chemistry.

• In Part I, you'll learn about all the factors that go into supporting—or disrupting—your metabolism: food, exercise, stress, sleep, and thyroid health.

• In Part II, you'll get a step-by-step guide for figuring out your own personal Plan. You'll lose a lot of weight in those 30 days—anywhere from 10 to 20 pounds—but even more important, you'll find out exactly what foods, exercise, sleep, and stress relief are right for you, so that you can keep losing weight easily.

• In Part III, you'll find out how to keep your Metabolism Plan working. You'll also learn how to tweak and adjust it as your circumstances and body change. That way you'll be set for the rest of your life.

When I tell my clients that they can eat what they want and enjoy what they eat, they often don't believe it. Yes, you can enjoy fried chicken, wine with dinner, a blowout birthday meal. Yes, you can eat "everything you want" as soon as you figure out what your body truly wants. Yes, you can cut back your exercise by a lot—maybe even to as little as 12 minutes a day, three days a week. Yes, when you do all these things, the weight comes off by itself, and you never have to think about it again.

"But that seems totally counterintuitive!" one of my clients told me. "How can I eat more—and lose weight? How can I exercise less—and lose weight? How can everything I've ever known about weight loss just be wrong?"

I get it. This probably does seem counterintuitive, because I'm telling you something that runs directly against all the dieting advice you've ever heard, read, or talked about with your friends. But it's 100 percent true, based on solid scientific research and years of working with clients who were never able to lose weight—until they came to me.

Think back to a time in your life when you were at your best, healthiest, most energized weight. I don't mean when you were exercising two hours a day or doing a juice cleanse—nobody can live like that, and nobody should have to. I mean a time when you were living normally and feeling great.

Well, we're going to get you back to that, and we're going to keep you there. We're going to win you the freedom to eat what you feel like eating and to exercise an amount that feels good while still maintaining a healthy weight. And if you never remember a time like that in your life, no worries. That time is coming soon.

So let's get started. I can't wait for you to enjoy all the benefits of your own personal Metabolism Plan!

Beth, Age 34

I've been on The Metabolism Plan for the past two months. I've lost 25 pounds, and I feel really *good* for the first time in years! My weight is now the least it has been in years, and I'm so excited. I have tried multiple programs over the years; I would get frustrated and quit because I wouldn't lose weight, and in some cases I even gained. Often, the programs made me feel crummy, too.

But on The Metabolism Plan, my blood sugars are under control for the first time in years. More importantly, I feel terrific! Well, at least until I deviate and eat "non-friendly" foods. One of the coolest things, though, is that when I get right back on my personalized regimen, I feel better quickly and the weight that I gained comes right back off.

One of the craziest things to me is that I am eating *tons* more calories than before, and yet the weight is still coming off. Most of the programs I tried over the years had me consuming around 1,200 calories a day and working out like a maniac, and yet they still didn't work. Until I found The Metabolism Plan, I had no idea how much I was starving my body. I now have a way of eating and exercising that makes sense to me, that works for me, and that I can be on for the rest of my life.

Part One

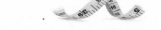

METABOLISM

YOUR KEY TO WEIGHT LOSS

CHAPTER ONE

The Metabolism Myth

Tanya, age 52, came to me at her wit's end. "I live on egg whites, salad, and salmon," she told me. "If I'm feeling really decadent, I have a few nuts as a snack or some berries for dessert. I do my workout as soon as I get home from work, and on weekends, I run five miles a day. But I'm always tired and always hungry. How can I eat so healthy and still be 50 pounds overweight? My doctors say I must be lying when I tell them what I eat. I think it's my thyroid, but they say my numbers are normal and that I just need to eat less and exercise more."

Naomi, 29, goes faithfully to the gym every day after work. "I never have dessert," she told me, almost in tears. "I never have bread or pasta or chips or carbs of any kind, really. Six days a week, I run on the treadmill, or go for a spin class. But every year, I keep gaining weight. What's wrong with me!"

Roberto has always eaten comfortably and exercised moderately, and for most of his life, his weight has been stable. In his late 40s, however, he gained 25 pounds, seemingly out of nowhere. When I ask him why he thinks he's suddenly having trouble, he doesn't know what to answer. As we continue to talk, though, he tells me that in the last few months, his wife has gotten laid off, his son was diagnosed with a learning disability, and his mother has entered a nursing home. His eating and exercise habits haven't changed—but his life has.

"I'm doing everything right—and yet, it's all going wrong."

These are the words I hear from my clients time and time again. They eat carefully—often too carefully, cutting out every trace of "fun food." They exercise vigorously—often too vigorously, stressing their bodies and pushing themselves too hard. Or maybe they skip exercise completely, believing that if they aren't able to give an hour a day, five days a week, their bodies won't respond at all. They often skimp on sleep and struggle with stress. Then they wonder why they can't lose those extra 10, 20, or 50 pounds. What exactly is going wrong?

If you can't lose weight—especially after following what you think is a healthy diet and exercise routine—there are basically two reasons:

- reactive foods
- metabolism.

So let's look at these two weight-loss culprits one by one to see just exactly how they are sabotaging your weight-loss efforts.

How Reactive Foods Cause Weight Gain

In the ideal world, you could eat just about any healthy food you can think of, and your body would respond appropriately. You'd digest that food, absorb its nutrients, and benefit from its contributions to your energy, well-being, and health.

However, for a number of reasons, we are not in that ideal world, and as a result, we often react to a particular food with an immune-system response known as *inflammation*. Inflammation is actually a healing process that can be tremendously helpful to your body as a short-term response to a specific infection or injury. However, when inflammation is triggered too often, it becomes chronic. And that's where the trouble begins.

In Chapter 4, you will learn exactly how certain foods can trigger inflammation, which in turn triggers weight gain. I call these inflammation triggers *reactive foods*, because your body is having an inflammatory reaction to them. They are a major culprit in weight gain, because even if you cut back on calories, exercise like a fiend, and otherwise "watch your weight," reactive foods can sabotage all your efforts.

Think that reactive foods are not your problem? Think again. Everyone I have ever met is eating at least three "healthy" foods that are inflammatory for them—not necessarily for everyone, but inflammatory for their unique biochemistry. That's why foods like spinach, tilapia, oatmeal, skim milk, asparagus, and cauliflower could be the issue behind your expanding waistline. The very foods you thought would keep you healthy and lean may be doing just the opposite.

Carrie, Age 34

Three years ago, I weighed 82 pounds more than I do today. I was starving from eating only 1,200 calories, exercising for an hour every day on my stationary bike, speed walking, and never sleeping. I couldn't take care of my baby—I was too heavy and too weak. Something had to change.

I saw Lyn-Genet on Fox News and began working with her. Her recipes were *nothing* like what I'd ever eaten, but I couldn't argue with her logic. I struggled through the cleanse and, to be honest, I didn't even make it all the way—on Day 3, I ate Triscuits like there was no tomorrow! But I learned that even when I eat reactive foods, I can get past it by eating foods that work for me the next day and the day after that. I can lose the little bit of weight I gained as long as I keep my inflammation down. And this is now a way of life for me.

There is no shortage of food on The Metabolism Plan—you eat till you're full. You learn how to watch your body for signs that a food is inflammatory for you, and by eliminating it you slowly figure out what foods work for you. Everyone is different. What works for you might not work for me. You might be able to eat bread and lose weight. I can't. I can't eat tomatoes, peppers, and paprika, either—if I eat even a small amount, the next day I'll be up a pound with swollen joints.

However, my body keeps changing. When I first started, I couldn't eat eggs without blowing up. Now, I can eat eggs every other day. By eliminating inflammatory foods, I allowed my body to heal—and I lost 97 pounds. I never dreamed I could get thinner than I was in college! And I can do so eating butter, avocados, sausage, and all kinds of foods that we've been told are "bad" for us—even chocolate and wine. Plus, I can do things I never thought I could do, like climb trees, run, and do cartwheels. I'm a new person!

I heartily recommend this approach to everyone, even if you're not overweight or only have a few pounds to lose. This doesn't just help people lose weight; it teaches a whole new way to become healthy. Do you have IBS? Acid reflux? Migraines? If you work with your body and study its reaction to food, you can learn to avoid the foods that create an inflammatory reaction. Many of our diseases today are the result of chronic inflammation. If we manage our inflammation, we can manage our diseases and reduce—even eliminate—our need for many medications.

I believe that most of us are chronically undernourished. We don't eat nutrient-dense foods, and we eat lots of processed junk. We ignore food sensitivities, unaware of the damage we are doing. The Metabolism Plan is one of the best tools to help you learn how to eat right for *your* body.

Besides weight gain, other mild inflammatory reactions include headache, skin issues, hormonal problems, mood swings, constipation, and bloating. Left untreated, chronic inflammation can cause far worse problems, including heart disease, type 2 diabetes, and even cancer.

A number of studies support the relationship between inflammation and chronic disease. For example, in the prestigious journal *Nature*, researchers Lisa M. Coussens and Zena Werb review the research on inflammation as a factor in the development of cancer. In their 2002 article "Inflammation and Cancer," they suggest that "inflammation is a critical component of tumour progression." In "The Linkage Between Inflammation and Type 2 Diabetes Mellitus," published in *Diabetes Research and Clinical Practice* in 2013, N.G. Cruz and colleagues assert that "inflammatory responses may have a role" in type 2 diabetes. These are just two of many, many articles pointing to the dangers of inflammation.

Can "healthy" foods really cause problems like that—foods like salmon, turkey, beans, and raw kale? You bet! Those foods may work wonderfully for your best friend. But if they are not right for *you*, they will provoke inflammation. And then you start to have issues. The good news—maybe even the great news—is that your reactive foods will stop causing you problems as soon as you cut them out.

Sometimes you might just need to eat certain foods less often. In my office, we say, "rotate or react"; that is, if you don't rotate your foods, you might start to produce a mild food sensitivity. For example, if you eat pizza and bagels every day, you can very easily become gluten intolerant, especially because pizza and bagels are so much higher in gluten than bread, pasta, and other baked goods. Stick to bread a few times a week, and you might be fine!

Do you have to give up the foods that are causing reactions forever? Probably not. On The Metabolism Plan, you'll have the chance to test every food that is important to you so you can find out whether it is inflammatory or healthy for you. When you discover foods that cause inflammatory reactions, you'll cut them out of your diet immediately. Then you will retest them in three months to a year to see when you can add them back in. It's very likely that you will be able to start eating them again without any issues at all.

How will you know which foods you can eat? That's the really terrific part of The Metabolism Plan: I'm not going to tell you what kind of diet you need to be on. Paleo, vegan, omnivore, whatever: It's your choice! All I want you to do is test the foods you love and see how your body responds to them. When you eat a food that causes inflammation, you'll gain weight the next day; if a food is good for your chemistry, you'll lose weight the next day. Either way, *you* are in charge of your metabolism and your weight.

Can you test fun foods, too? Sure, you can even test Scotch if you want to! Instead of feeling that all your indulgences are off-limits, you'll discover that many can be a regular part of your diet, and some can be a semi-regular part of your diet—all without you gaining permanent weight or triggering other health issues.

Cecile, Age 39

My favorite thing about The Metabolism Plan is that it doesn't dictate what I can and can't eat. Instead, it's a way of discovering what does and doesn't work for my body. If I decide to indulge in a not-so-friendly food, the next day I can stick to my friendly food list and minimize the effects. It's amazing to me that more doctors and nutritionists are not recommending this to *all* of their patients.

Oatmeal, peanut butter, and all the health foods I had been eating to lose weight were unfriendly to me, causing me to gain weight and irritate my colitis symptoms. White bread, pancakes, lamb, even cupcakes—all foods I was told to avoid—are foods that I can eat with no problems, and that help me lose weight! It's really incredible and I am thankful every day that I found this way of eating.

But reactive foods are only one part of the problem. The other is your metabolism, so let's take a look at that.

How Your Metabolism Can Cause Weight Gain

How do you feel about your metabolism? Maybe you're envious of friends who have a "fast metabolism" and seem to eat whatever they want without gaining an ounce. Maybe you worry that your own metabolism is "slow" because you seem to gain 2 pounds just looking at a cookie.

Well, guess what? Whatever you think about your metabolism, you are going to find out how to boost your metabolic function so that you can lose weight while enjoying delicious foods and devoting only a little time each week to exercise. To get these fabulous results, though, you need to understand what your metabolism is and how it works.

Your metabolism is a set of chemical transformations that takes place within your body to transform the food you eat into your bones, blood, muscles, organs, nerves, and biochemicals, as well as into the energy that sustains you. Your metabolism determines how hungry you are, how often you need or want to eat, and how much food you need to sustain you. It also determines whether you gain, lose, or maintain weight, as well as how much energy you have.

In a perfectly healthy body, your metabolism continually maintains a healthy weight, seemingly without effort. Keeping your body at an optimal weight is meant to be an easy task, something that your body does as simply as breathing.

However, when your metabolic function is disrupted, your body will put on weight that it absolutely refuses to let go. In fact, the harder you try to lose weight—the less you eat, the more you exercise, the harder you push yourself—the more your body will dig in and hold on to weight. Your body is sending you a very clear message: "What you're doing is not working."

Getting to this point can be such a painful experience. You start to feel like there is something wrong with you. You wonder why everyone else seems to lose weight so easily. You can't help asking yourself, "What's wrong with *me?*"

Well, I am here to tell you that nothing is wrong with you. You are perfect. And so is your body, which is speaking to you every day, trying to tell you what it needs. The only problem is that you don't yet have the tools to understand what your body is saying. Once you finish this book, you will have those tools, and you'll be able to see just how perfect you are!

So what's disrupting your metabolism? Here are the major factors.

- **Reactive foods**: As we just saw, when you eat foods that provoke inflammation, you almost inevitably provoke weight gain as well. That's the issue we focused on in *The Plan,* and it's a common problem—maybe even the most common reason behind weight and health issues. But there are others, which this book will also help you take care of.
- **Thyroid**: Your thyroid gland produces thyroid hormone, the fuel that powers your cells while regulating metabolic function. When your thyroid function is disrupted, your metabolism is disrupted, too, and you gain weight or aren't able to lose it. Until your thyroid gets the support it needs—the right nutrients, sufficient sleep, and adequate stress relief—you are most likely to be facing weight issues.

    I don't want to worry you, but you probably have a thyroid problem without even realizing it. Sad but true: Many people with thyroid issues have not been properly diagnosed, and many more have been diagnosed but are not getting the proper treatment they need. You'll learn more about this in Chapter 2, but meanwhile, do *not* assume this aspect of metabolism does not apply to you. It might very well be the source of all your weight issues.

Abe, Age 52

I have tried for more than 20 years to lose weight. I went through every weight-loss and gym program you can imagine. I would lose a few pounds, and then it would all come to a standstill. Every nutritionist and trainer I saw would ask me the same question, "Are you sure you are following the program?"

Then I found out through a friend about The Metabolism Plan. All those years I had been eating foods that I was supposed to—foods like quinoa, shrimp, and protein shakes—thinking I was doing what was right. Now I know that I am reactive to those foods.

I started working with a trainer who's a Metabolism Planner, and now I actually have a six-pack. Best of all, I've lost more than 36 pounds!

- **Stress**: Stress disrupts your thyroid as well as other aspects of your metabolism. A certain amount of stress is stimulating and energizing, but chronic stress can play havoc with your metabolism and therefore with your weight.
- **Sleep**: Lack of sleep is a form of stress that disrupts both your thyroid and endocrine system, leaving you with a sluggish metabolism that makes it nearly impossible to lose weight.
- **Exercise**: Believe it or not, exercise can also be a form of stress when it challenges your body too much. The right type of exercise can help you lose weight, relieve stress, and rev up your metabolism to optimal levels. However, the wrong type of exercise can disrupt your metabolism and sabotage your weight-loss efforts.

The good news is that once you understand what's going on with food, thyroid, stress, and exercise, you can support your metabolism rather than disrupt it. But first things first. Let's look at all the myths about metabolism and clear them up, one by one, so that you truly understand what your metabolism needs.

Michael, Age 46

Between a hectic work schedule and the desires to be a good dad and husband, I don't have the time or interest in dieting, but I do care a lot about my health. I'm also an amateur triathlete, so fitness and energy levels matter a lot. Lyn doesn't tell me how to diet; she helps me figure out the best foods to eat to promote a healthy, energetic state of being. Her approach is strictly tailored to me—both in evaluating what foods make my body happy and in providing the encouragement and nutritional science behind why my body acts the way it does. She's so much fun and easy to work with. But best of all, I can look and feel better!

MYTH 1: I'M EATING ALL THE RIGHT FOODS, SO I SHOULD BE ABLE TO LOSE WEIGHT.

FACT: SOME "RIGHT" FOODS ARE VERY, VERY WRONG.

You probably wouldn't be surprised if eating a diet full of processed foods or high in dietary sugars would cause weight gain. But what if, like Tanya, you're living on egg whites, salads, and salmon? What if, like Naomi, you've ruthlessly cut carbs out of your diet, never allowing yourself a single indulgence?

Well, apart from the fact that these kinds of restrictions are depressing, there's another problem:

Many supposedly "healthy" foods may not work for your chemistry.

These foods may be perfectly healthy for somebody else—but for you (and thousands like you), they are what I call "reactive." That is, as we have seen, they provoke your immune system to produce inflammation, which causes immediate weight gain.

How is this possible? It starts with *histamine*, which causes your *capillaries* to dilate. Capillaries are your tiniest blood vessels, and they respond to changes in fluid very quickly. When these dilated capillaries leak fluid into your tissue, your weight goes up immediately.

But this causes an inflammatory response that does not just cause water weight. (A shame, because water weight can be reversed within a day.) It also kick-starts any health issues you might have: constipation, acid reflux, irritable bowel syndrome (IBS), arthritis, migraines, and so on, in an inflammatory response that can last up to 72 hours.

To control this response, your body produces a stress hormone known as *cortisol.* Cortisol has many functions, and we'll learn more about it throughout this book. For now, let me just tell you that cortisol uses the same biochemical building blocks as several other key hormones, including progesterone and testosterone. So the more cortisol your body produces, the more your hormones are thrown out of whack, disrupting your water balance, metabolism, thyroid health, sex drive, and immune response. To make matters worse, elevated cortisol levels also trigger increased glucose, which leads to elevated blood sugar.

So now we have a new set of problems, because when your blood sugar goes up, it feeds a type of intestinal bacteria known as *yeast*, or *candida.* Intestinal yeast has specialized glucose sensors, enabling it to zero in on this new supply of sugar. That's great for them, but not so good for you, because that hungry yeast alters your gut flora—the bacterial population that lives in your gut and helps promote digestion, a healthy immune system, and a number of other bodily functions. Since 70 to 80 percent of your immune system is located in your gut, you're now looking at a disrupted immune response as well as digestive dysfunction, skin problems, hormonal issues, chronic pain, autoimmune disease, depression, brain fog, and anxiety. A high yeast population also means never-ending carb and sugar cravings. Long term, you're at risk for obesity and diabetes.

Every single time you eat a food that doesn't work for *you*, this whole process begins. And that is why it's so vital for you to do The Metabolism Plan: It's not just your weight; it's your health.

We'll look more closely at inflammation in Chapter 4. For now, take a look at the following reactive foods list and see if some of your go-to weight-loss foods are on it—foods are listed in order of the percentage of people who react to them. If you find them, you've just learned part of the reason you are struggling with weight and symptoms.

REACTIVE FOODS

85%+ Reactive
- Asparagus
- Bagels
- Black beans
- Cabbage
- Cannellini beans
- Cauliflower
- Corn
- Deli meats (regular sodium)
- Eggplant
- Farm-raised fish
- Greek yogurt
- Hard-boiled eggs
- Non-organic spinach
- Oatmeal
- Raspberries
- Salmon
- Shrimp
- Strawberries
- Sushi with sauces
- Tomato sauce
- Turkey
- Veal

70% Reactive
- Bananas
- Green beans
- Green peppers
- Pasta
- Pineapple
- Roasted nut butter
- Tofu
- Walnuts
- Yogurt, regular

60% Reactive
- Artichokes
- Cod
- Grapefruit
- Mahimahi
- Melon (except watermelon)
- Mushrooms (excluding shiitake)

60% Reactive (cont.)
- Oranges
- Pork
- Quinoa
- Red peppers
- Tahini
- Tuna

50% Reactive
- Almond milk
- Couscous
- Cow's milk
- Edamame
- Tomatoes
- White rice
- Whole eggs

40% Reactive
- Brussels sprouts
- Lactose-free milk
- Pinto beans
- Whole eggs

30% Reactive
- Bok choy
- Cow's cheese
- Egg whites
- Flounder
- Halibut
- Lentils
- Scallops

20% Reactive
- Bread
- Butternut squash
- Crab
- Fennel
- Snow peas
- Watermelon

15% Reactive
- Amaranth
- Kamut
- Spelt

10% Reactive
- Chickpeas
- Duck
- Hemp seeds
- Potatoes

5% or less reactive
- Apples
- Avocado
- Basmati rice
- Beef
- Beets
- Blueberries
- Broccoli
- Carrots
- Chia seeds
- Chicken
- Coconut milk
- Endive
- Frisée
- Garlic
- Goat or sheep's cheese
- Kale
- Lamb
- Leeks
- Mango
- Onions
- Pears
- Pumpkin seeds
- Radicchio
- Raw almonds
- Rice milk
- Shiitake mushrooms (may be higher if you have yeast)
- Sunflower seeds
- Yellow squash
- Zucchini

You'll learn more about the "healthy eating trap" in Chapter 4. And during your 30 days on The Metabolism Plan, you'll have the chance to test foods so you can find out exactly which ones are reactive for you. Maybe you've been choosing a "healthy" turkey burger and mashed cauliflower, only to discover that those foods are making you fat and sick, and you would have been just fine with a cheeseburger and fries. Maybe yogurt doesn't work for you—but fried calamari does. Maybe salsa is your enemy but guacamole is your friend. Won't it be a relief to find out once and for all which foods cause you to gain weight and which you can safely enjoy?

MYTH 2: MY METABOLISM NATURALLY SLOWS DOWN AS I GET OLDER.

FACT: THANK GOODNESS, NO. AGE IS NOT THE PROBLEM—FUNCTION IS.

This is such a widespread, durable myth that I'll give you the truth loud and clear: *Your metabolism does not naturally slow down as you get older.* At least, it doesn't have to. What does happen as you age is that your thyroid function is more affected by hormonal fluctuations, and your digestive function starts to slow down. This process is amplified by a lifetime of eating reactive foods and perhaps also the wrong types of exercise combined with excess stress.

So once again, there's quite a bit of good news: As soon as you start eating and exercising in the ways that are right for you, your thyroid levels balance, your digestion improves, and your metabolism can rev up to your teenage levels—or beyond. I've even had clients go to their middle-school weight!

Think of these next 30 days as your own personal investigation into your metabolism. What kinds of foods, exercise, sleep, and stress relief does your body like? When you know the answers, you can give your body what it wants. Your body will reward you with a healthy weight, great mood, tons of energy, and glowing good health.

MYTH 3: I CAN'T HAVE A THYROID PROBLEM—EITHER
I'VE TESTED NORMAL OR I'M CURRENTLY ON THE
RIGHT DOSE OF THYROID HORMONE.

FACT: AT LEAST 30 MILLION AMERICANS HAVE
THYROID DYSFUNCTION AND MILLIONS MORE ARE
UNDIAGNOSED.

Let me give it to you straight. If you want to lose weight and can't, if
you want to lose weight and can only do so with an enormous amount
of effort, or if you seem to be "mysteriously" gaining weight, it's almost
a sure bet that your thyroid is involved. A staggering number of Americans have thyroid issues without even realizing it. So many of my clients come into my office in tears over weight issues, never realizing
that their weight problem is fundamentally a thyroid problem.

But it's more than just weight, because you can have thyroid dysfunction even at your perfect weight! Thyroid problems can mean
that you have no energy and no sex drive. You're constipated and
moody. Your hair is falling out and your digestion is rotten. You can't
focus and your memory seems to be completely gone.

Once you give your thyroid the support it needs, though, that can
all change. Overnight.

The chances that you have a thyroid problem go up exponentially
if you are a woman over the age of 40 because for us, thyroid issues
are a veritable epidemic. And guess what? Obesity in that population
has also reached epidemic proportions. And yes, there is a connection.

Here's a fact that I find really upsetting: Even if you've been tested
for thyroid problems and your tests come back "normal," you may
still have a thyroid problem. So your doctor says you're fine—but you
keep gaining weight.

To make matters worse, the problems don't end even when you
are prescribed some thyroid medication, because you might easily be
getting the wrong type of thyroid hormone or a dose that is too low.
That's beyond frustrating: It looks as though you are being correctly

treated, but your thyroid is still underfunctioning and your metabolism is still out of whack. So the weight problems continue, no matter how you tinker with diet and exercise. Your doctor might tell you that everything is fine—but your body knows better.

You'll learn more about your thyroid in Chapter 2. And when you start your 30 days, you'll test for the best ways to support your thyroid, so that it is finally able to operate at peak efficiency and your metabolism can return to normal. A lot of other symptoms will probably disappear along with the unwanted weight: constipation, skin problems, memory issues, anxiety…the list goes on and on.

MYTH 4: IF I HAVE THYROID PROBLEMS, MEDICATION IS ENOUGH TO SOLVE THEM.

FACT: WHILE YOU MIGHT NEED MEDS, YOUR DIET, EXERCISE LEVELS, SLEEP PATTERNS, AND STRESS LEVELS ALL HAVE A HUGE IMPACT ON YOUR THYROID.

If medication were enough to solve your thyroid problems, my office wouldn't be filled with clients who are overweight, exhausted, depressed, and lacking a sex drive! Medication is simply not enough to make you feel 100 percent.

The great news? Going on The Metabolism Plan may be able to help you decrease your medication. The exciting thing about the 30-day journey ahead is that you'll find out which foods and lifestyle your thyroid needs, making it stronger and more functional.

MYTH 5: HOW MUCH I SLEEP HAS NOTHING TO DO WITH MY WEIGHT.

FACT: SLEEP IS A KEY FACTOR IN EITHER SUPPORTING OR DISRUPTING YOUR METABOLISM.

Your body needs time to rest and repair. In fact, that's when you can lose the most weight! I know you might be able to *get by* on six hours of sleep, but for every two hours of sleep you don't get, your weight loss is impaired, anywhere from 0.2 pound to more than a pound. See for yourself how much extra weight you can lose on those Saturdays and Sundays when you get to sleep in or when you cut out those 5:30 a.m. boot camps.

MYTH 6: THE MORE I EXERCISE, THE MORE WEIGHT I CAN LOSE.

FACT: YOU NEED TO EXERCISE AT THE RIGHT LEVEL FOR *YOU*. IF YOU GET MORE EXERCISE THAN YOUR BODY NEEDS, YOU PUT YOURSELF AT RISK FOR WEIGHT GAIN.

I've seen it with thousands of clients, and with myself as well: Too much exercise raises cortisol, which cues your body to gain weight. Learning how to do the right amount of exercise—but not too much—is key to weight loss.

That's because when you relieve stress—including physical stress, like intense exercise—you lose more weight. It's a crucial point, and one of the reasons The Metabolism Plan is going to change your world.

MYTH 7: IT'S GOOD TO EXERCISE EVERY DAY.

FACT: PROBABLY NOT. FOR ALMOST EVERYBODY, THE OPTIMAL EXERCISE PATTERN IS EVERY OTHER DAY.

Why? Because exercise is a two-part process. First, you exercise... then you rest and repair so that your body can restore itself on a higher level. Exercise, restore; exercise, restore. That's the way you achieve peak physical fitness, a healthy weight, and a metabolism that runs efficiently.

Some people do benefit from daily training, and I'll tell you how to figure out whether you are one of those people. You might just be genetically gifted—a natural athlete who benefits from a daily workout.

For most of us, though, every day is too often, especially as we age and our body begins to repair itself more slowly. The accumulated inflammation of many years might also take its toll, especially if other stressors in our life are on high. So just about all of us need a repair day after an exercise "stress" day. In fact, if you exercise too frequently, your body will perceive this as additional stress and start *gaining* weight in response. So in the next 30 days, you're going to test how often, how long, and how intensely to exercise, so you can be sure your workout routines are exactly right for you.

MYTH 8: WALKING 30 OR MORE MINUTES A DAY WILL HELP ME LOSE WEIGHT.

FACT: SORRY, BUT HIGHLY UNLIKELY.

Kick that Fitbit to the curb! Walking is not the greatest exercise for most people, so let me lay it out for you.

If you are completely unused to physical activity, walking is probably a good choice for you to get back into some kind of movement. Walking 20 to 30 minutes a day at a brisk pace can be an effective form of exercise for you, just until you get in shape.

However, once you *are* in shape, walking won't be enough of a challenge to count as exercise. Your body will quickly adapt to walking and the weight loss will stop. Yet if you walk *more* than 30 minutes, your body might perceive walking as stress…and stress cues your body to gain weight. In fact, some of my folks who have the hardest time with weight loss are the ones who take their dogs on long walks!

I know a lot of people are very attached to walking, and if you are one of those folks, don't panic. I'll help you find the balance that works for you so you can figure out how much walking is too much while still keeping your puppies happy.

MYTH 9: I HAVE NO WILLPOWER.

FACT: YOU DO! YOUR FOOD CRAVINGS AREN'T A LACK OF CONTROL. THEY ARE PHYSIOLOGICAL REACTIONS TO STRESS AND INFLAMMATORY FOODS.

Cravings are *not* about control. They are usually due to factors that you would never guess play a huge part in your 4 p.m. snacks or midnight cravings—hormones and inflammation. As soon as you know how to moderate stress and avoid reactive foods, you'll be amazed at how your cravings evaporate.

Meanwhile, please don't believe those ugly myths about yourself—that you have no self-control, that your health and weight issues are your own fault because you lack discipline. It's not about willpower; it's just basic biology. Your body *wants* to get to a healthy weight. And getting there is so much easier than you think.

Loving Your Metabolism

Nothing makes me sadder than to hear a client say, "I've got a terrible metabolism." Your metabolism is ready to operate at peak function—you just need to support it through the choices that are right for you. It's not your fault that you haven't known what your body needs—but now you will! So let's start by looking at the gland that regulates your metabolism, governs your energy, and helps determine your weight: your thyroid.

Lila, Age 33

I have always had digestive issues. I was the kid at the table who wouldn't eat—I'd just mash my food around to make it look like I made a dent in it. My mom would always ask me, "How old are you?" If I said, "Ten years old," she would reply, "Then you need to take ten more bites." Every year on my birthday I would blow out the candles and think . . . ugh another year, another bite.

Things got worse around senior year of high school when food started making me really sick. I would get horrible heartburn, bloating, cramping, and diarrhea. This was the start of my journey to try to figure out what was wrong with my digestion as I started cutting out foods. The first to go was orange juice, then chocolate, then soda, then tomato sauce, then all fruit . . . and so on.

Since then, I have been to more doctors than I could name and no one seemed to know what was wrong with me, nor did they seem to care. I was diagnosed with IBS, acid reflux, small intestinal bacterial overgrowth, Crohn's disease, and colitis. After years of taking medication after medication, I stopped them all at age 29. Then I started gaining weight despite not changing my eating habits, until at 33 I had gained 35 pounds and felt the worst I have ever felt in my life.

That's when a friend told me about The Metabolism Plan and I started working with Lyn-Genet. The first day of the cleanse I lost 6 pounds. I thought it was a mistake! But I looked in the mirror, and it looked like someone had taken a pin and popped me. So I kept it up, and by the end of the cleanse I had lost 10 pounds.

Now, after following Lyn-Genet's approach, for the first time in over 20 years, I do not have that pain in my stomach every day. My autoimmune disease is healing purely through eating the right food for my body, rather than following a cookie-cutter, one-size-fits-all diet. I am back at work, and I feel great. It's taken me a long time to get here, but the rough road has only made me stronger and helped me appreciate the good things in life all the more.

- -

CHAPTER TWO

Your Thyroid and Your Metabolism: What Your Doctor Won't Tell You

Your thyroid is basically your body's metabolic CEO. Like many bosses, it can be very temperamental, demanding your complete compliance. And like an unhappy boss, an unhappy thyroid can make your life a misery.

However, once you set up a good working relationship based on a good understanding of what your thyroid needs, you are golden. Give your thyroid the food, exercise, and sleep that it requires, and sooner than you ever thought possible, you and your metabolism will be set for life. The rewards are amazing—your thyroid's equivalent of a big promotion and a huge year-end bonus:

- Your weight comes off easily and stays off.
- You've got all the energy you could ever want, and then some!
- Your sex life is humming along in peak condition, and everything works the way it's supposed to. (Yes, that goes for both men and women!)
- Your digestion functions smoothly: no nausea, bloating, constipation, or diarrhea.

- Your mind is sharp and clear, your memory is excellent, and your focus is superb.
- Your mood is calm and balanced: no mood swings, depression, or anxiety.

Are you having trouble believing that your thyroid gland—a part of your body you probably haven't given much thought to—can do all that? Well, yes. It can! So let me introduce you to your thyroid gland, because in just 30 days, your grouchy metabolic boss is going to become your new best friend.

Thyroid Biology 101: Meet Your New Best Friend

The thyroid is a tiny gland located at the base of your throat. It's made of two lobes and is shaped like a butterfly. It weighs only about an ounce. Yet this minuscule gland has the power to make or break your metabolism.

Why is the thyroid so powerful? Partly because every cell in your body has receptors for thyroid hormones. That means that without just the right amount of those hormones, none of your cells can function properly.

Your thyroid is also responsible for the speed of your metabolism; it's the internal regulator that keeps everything on track for your best health and weight. So anything we can do to keep your thyroid in a happy place means that you will feel and look your best.

How Your Thyroid Works

Don't worry—we're not getting into a heavy science lesson here! But I do want you to visualize how everything works so you can give your thyroid the resources it needs to support you.

Your thyroid gland is part of a complex system that's supposed to keep your thyroid hormone at just the right level. It all starts with the hypothalamus, which you can think of as "command central" as it keeps watch over your hormone levels. The moment you are about to run low on thyroid hormone, your hypothalamus sets thyroid production in motion via a biochemical known as *thyrotropin-releasing hormone (TRH)*.

TRH in turn triggers your pituitary, a small gland at the base of your brain. Your pituitary produces its own special chemical—*thyroid-stimulating hormone*, or TSH—which, appropriately enough, stimulates your thyroid. These three glands together make up the *hypothalamus-pituitary-thyroid axis*.

I want you to remember TSH, because if your doctor ever tests you for thyroid issues, TSH is probably the first thing they will measure. When the TSH reaches your thyroid, it prods that gland into action, causing it to produce several types of thyroid hormone—most importantly, T4 and T3. Here's how it works.

> T4 is the inactive form of thyroid hormone and it converts into the metabolic powerhouse T3. Whenever your body needs more power, T4 converts into more T3. Having T4 in your bloodstream is another way your body keeps thyroid hormone at the right level. Having optimal T3 levels means you're at peak functioning. When your hypothalamus-pituitary-thyroid axis is working perfectly, the thyroid hormone in your blood always remains at the right level. Picture a continuous feedback loop (see page 25):

That's what's *supposed* to happen. However, a number of different factors can disrupt this process and dysregulate your thyroid, keeping it from producing the right level of hormones. And, my friends, that can spell trouble.

What Disrupts Your Thyroid?

- Reactive foods—that is, the wrong foods for your body
- The wrong exercise for your body

- An imbalance in other hormones, including estrogen, progesterone, and testosterone
- Not enough good sleep
- Too much stress
- Nutritional deficiencies

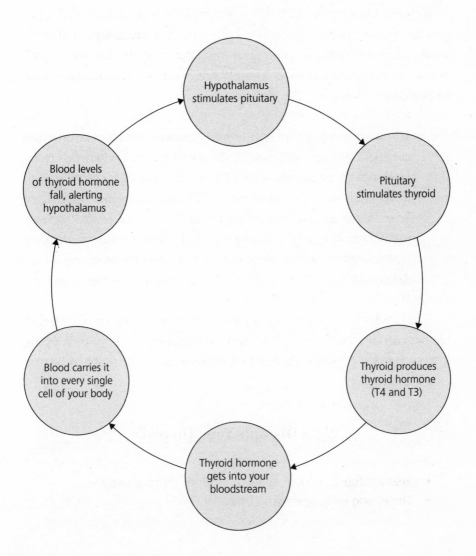

When any of these factors affect your thyroid, your thyroid hormone is likely to be at the wrong level. You can become *hypothyroid* (your thyroid hormone levels are too low) or *hyperthyroid* (your thyroid hormone levels are too high). You might also start to suffer from other thyroid-related disorders.

For example, a number of studies have shown that over-exercise can suppress thyroid function. In 2003, the *European Journal of Applied Physiology* published an article showing that intense, prolonged exercise training could suppress TSH and free T3 in female college athletes who engaged in such daily exercise as rowing, running, and weight lifting. In 2005, a study published in *Neuroendocrinology Letters* found that intense aerobic exercise could cause a drop in both overall and free T3 levels.

In other words, the right levels of exercise can be terrific for your thyroid, but overdoing it disrupts your thyroid function and slows your metabolism. Luckily, all the factors that suppress thyroid function are things you can have control over. You can eat "friendly" foods and avoid "unfriendly" ones (see Chapter 4). You can exercise the way and amount that works best for you (see Chapter 5). You can bring your other hormones into balance, and you can get night after night of restful sleep, allowing your body optimal repair.

And now that you know about these factors, you are one step closer to mastering your metabolism!

Who Is at Higher Risk for Earlier Thyroid Issues?

• **Vegetarians and vegans**: Many of the nutrients needed to support optimal thyroid health, such as B12, aren't plentiful enough in vegetarian or vegan diets. Plus, these diets tend toward an over-reliance on proteins like soy. A 2011 study found that supplementing with soy phytoestrogens resulted in a threefold increase in the risk of developing hypothyroidism. Animal studies have also found a link between soy and thyroid dysfunction. Moreover, many fruits and vegetables can attack thyroid function as well. These so-called *goitrogens* (attackers of thyroid) include cauliflower, spinach, strawberries, and swiss chard. Now, have I taught my vegetarian and vegan clients how to have great thyroid health? Absolutely yes, so if you are in this category, don't worry: You'll learn everything you need to do to keep that metabolism revved to full blast.

• **Athletes**: Exercising beyond the threshold that is right for your body can deplete your body of nutrients. Over-exercise can also attack the production of T3 and the conversion of T4 into T3. It's as though your body gets worried that you're expending too much energy and tries to slow you down. Again, the solution is simple: Test how exercise affects your body (which you'll learn how to do in the next 30 days) and stick to what's right for you.

Hypothyroidism: When Your Thyroid Under-Performs

Hypothyroidism results when your thyroid gland fails to produce enough hormone. New research shows that this condition can be induced by a number of factors such as stress, over-exercise, hormonal imbalance, or nutritional deficiencies. Most notably, a 2005 study published in *Thyroid Journal Program* outlines how stress negatively affects immune response, leading to thyroid dysfunction and autoimmune thyroid disorders, and research published in *Current Sports Medicine Reports* in 2009 shows that over-exercise lowers T3 and T4 levels in athletes.

The most common form of hypothyroidism is an autoimmune disorder known as Hashimoto's thyroiditis. Like other autoimmune disorders, Hashimoto's occurs when your immune system produces antibodies that attack your own tissue.

Now, since 70 percent of your immune system is located in your gut, immune problems are closely related to gut function, as a whole body of research affirms. So as you can see, folks, it's all related:

poor gut function → dysfunctional immune system → disordered thyroid → sluggish metabolism

The solution? Heal your gut and repair gut function, and both your immune system and your thyroid will be a whole lot happier. You can take a big step in that direction by avoiding the reactive foods that disrupt gut function in the first place.

What Else Can Cause Hypothyroidism?

- Thyroid surgery (thyroidectomy) removes all or a large portion of your thyroid gland and thereby halts or diminishes hormone production.
- Radiation therapy used to treat cancers of the head and neck can also affect your thyroid gland and might lead to hypothyroidism.

Rachel, Age 43

In 2011, I came to Lyn-Genet feeling lost and confused. Why was I, a professional personal trainer with a degree in fitness, weighing 170 pounds? Why did everything I ate make me feel bloated and sick? I was ready to try a new approach, because my current one sure wasn't working!

In the first 30 days working with Lyn-Genet, I lost 30 pounds! Under her concerned and watchful eye, we discovered that I had been eating *all* the wrong things. Because at that time I didn't know how to cook, my daily eating in restaurants was also sending my sodium levels through the roof!

Now I enjoy cooking for myself and others. I've realized that anytime I crave something "easy," like a burger, I can make it for myself at home, with less salt and therefore less weight gain. (For an explanation of how salt causes weight gain, see page 73.)

My attitude toward food has become a healthy one. I enjoy eating to feel good, my body appreciates it, and I'm definitely not sacrificing taste. Thanks to Lyn-Genet, I'm much more educated about food, and I'm also able to be more insightful and educational when it comes to my clients' needs.

Sometimes your gut needs a little extra boost. I have found that many people benefit from a six-week dose of a supplement called MSM, which helps your gut lining to heal. Also beneficial is a *probiotic*—a capsule, liquid, or powder that contains billions of healthy bacteria, to repopulate the friendly bacteria that your gut needs for optimal function. Together, MSM and probiotics can help restore good digestion, ease inflammation, and promote weight loss.

How Do You Know if You Are Hypothyroid?

You may have or experience one or more of the following:

- Low energy
- Depression
- Constantly feeling cold
- Constipation
- Poor nail and hair growth
- Weight gain
- High cholesterol
- Hormonal disorders and lowered sex drive.

Hyperthyroidism: When Your Thyroid Over-Performs

Sometimes your thyroid produces too much thyroid hormone, a condition known as *hyperthyroidism*. This can occur for a number of reasons:

- Graves' disease is a type of autoimmune disorder in which antibodies produced by your immune system overstimulate your thyroid. Research such as the extensive studies listed in the 2011 journal *Cellular & Molecular Immunology* explains that autoimmune diseases are related to gut function, so when we bring down inflammation and heal gut function, we can go a long way toward healing autoimmune disease. That's why I recommend MSM and probiotics for Graves' as well as for Hashimoto's. While there are no permanent cures for auto-immune disorders, maintaining good gut function and low inflammation can keep them in remission.

- Hyperfunctioning thyroid nodules such as an adenoma (a benign tumor in your thyroid) can cause overproduction of thyroid hormone.
- Excess iodine can overstimulate your thyroid.
- Thyroiditis, or inflammation of the thyroid gland, can lead to either under- or over-performance of your thyroid gland.
- Tumors of the ovaries or testes can trigger hyperthyroidism.
- Too high a dose of thyroid medication can cause your thyroid to overproduce.

How Do You Know if You Are Hyperthyroid?

You may have or experience:

- Irritability
- Hair loss
- Anxiety
- Inability to sleep
- Heart palpitations
- Sudden weight loss
- Trembling of fingers
- Digestive issues
- Enlarged goiter
- Bulging eyes.

Thyroid and Your Mood

There is an unholy alliance between anxiety, depression, and your thyroid. I want you to feel better, so listen carefully: Many mood disorders can be resolved when your thyroid is functional. My mother suffered from chronic depression, so I know very well how debilitating that can be—how it can wreck your life and the lives of those who love you. I don't want you to go through what she did, and I certainly don't want to see you suffering. Something as simple as eating foods that suit your chemistry can frequently resolve decades of depression or anxiety. When using The Metabolism Plan and working with their medical team, many of my clients have been able to wean themselves off their antidepressants, and this might well be possible for you, too. You owe it to yourself to support your thyroid so you, too, can feel better! (Always be sure to work with your doctor if you want to change your dosage or stop any medication.)

Besides depression, hypothyroidism usually means you are struggling with low energy, weight gain, constipation, and difficulty concentrating. Hyperthyroidism can produce the same cognitive issues but tends to provoke more insomnia, irritability, and anxiety. In both cases, a dysfunctional thyroid can cause moodiness or mood swings.

The good news is, you can fix this. When you find what works for your body, your body will do what it always wants to do: heal. And when you see how badly your body wants to heal, and how quickly it can do so, you are back in the best relationship of your life—with yourself.

Thyroid and Cholesterol

Did you know that your high cholesterol might be due to an imbalance in your thyroid? I find that as soon as the thyroid starts to function properly, cholesterol can drop 40 to 60 points. I've even seen a 100-point drop and a newly balanced lipid panel in as little as 40 days! An article published in February 2016 in the physicians' resource

UpToDate reviewed the relationship between hypothyroidism, cholesterol, and cardiovascular disease, citing some 50 studies on the topic. Generally, research found a strong association between thyroid under-performance and high cholesterol.

Mariam, Age 41

After "eating clean" on The Metabolism Plan and jogging with my neighbor for the first time in my life, I have finally seen improvement! I have lost 13 pounds. I've achieved my real goal of lowering my cholesterol. And I am forever grateful! Check out my cholesterol results comparing today (my 41st birthday) and 9 months ago:

- Total cholesterol fell from 235 to 180, a drop of 55 points.
- LDL (bad cholesterol) fell from 183 to 123, a drop of 60 points.
- Triglycerides fell from 70 to 53.
- HDL (good cholesterol) remains steady at 47.

Al, Age 59

For most of my adult life, my weight has ranged from 165 to 185, mostly in the 180 range. My cholesterol level has consistently been on the high side (250 to 280) except for a few periods when I actively worked to lose weight, which I could only do temporarily. For the past few years, I thought that careful eating and moderate exercise could help me maintain a lower weight and lower my cholesterol. However, I remained stuck, and I was growing concerned that the trend was going in the wrong direction.

The Metabolism Plan appeared to provide a clear path forward. After 20 days, I lost 15 pounds and my cholesterol and lipid levels dropped dramatically:

Blood Chemistry Data

Measure	Pre–Metabolism Plan	Post–Metabolism Plan
Total Cholesterol	250	197
Triglycerides	142	78
HDL	48	53
LDL	174	128

I work full-time in an administrative position and I am expected to participate in numerous lunches, dinners, and receptions. I do my best to select friendly foods, and I've found that I can remain successful. The cholesterol results, the weight loss, and the general feeling of well-being have made me a passionate supporter of The Metabolism Plan.

I feel great, and I continue to maintain my weight loss. My overall eating patterns have changed, and I can quickly recover when I make other choices. It's a bonus that I get to have wine, cheese, and chocolate daily! Thanks, Lyn-Genet!

It's a Woman's Thing—Or Is It?

Women are vastly more likely to suffer from thyroid dysfunction at an earlier age than men—which, if you've been wondering, is a big part of the reason why women tend to gain weight more quickly than men, and why we have a harder time keeping it off.

Part—okay, most—of the issue is our blessed female hormones. If you're a woman, the fluctuations that you undergo each month from puberty to menopause set you up to have thyroid issues sooner than men.

But, men, you are not off the hook. You start to catch up with us as you age. Some of that is because your testosterone levels drop, and so do your levels of a chemical known as HGH (human growth hormone), which keeps your body growing and replenishing its cells, and whose levels tend to drop as you get older.

Another age-related issue for both men and women is that our glands tend to shrink as we age, including the thyroid gland. As a result, we have access to lower levels of thyroid hormone.

Don't worry—aging doesn't doom you to a future of excess weight, thinning hair, constipation, and brain fog. You can fight back with the right diet, supplements, exercise, and sleep. The first step is awareness—which is why you're reading this chapter, right?

Higher-risk men can develop thyroid issues as early as their 30s. Others begin having problems in their late 40s, and it just keeps going from there. By their late 50s, 70 percent of all men have some form of thyroid irregularity.

Here's the rotten part: Because thyroid issues are thought of as a woman's disease, men are often not tested appropriately, nor are their results scrutinized as deeply. This sets you up for failure, guys—or at least, it did so until now. Make sure to ask your doctor for a full thyroid panel if you note any of the symptoms in the lists on pages 29 and 30.

Hormones and Your Thyroid

The three primary sex hormones are estrogen, progesterone, and testosterone. Both men and women have some of each, although obviously, the proportions are different. When you have too much estrogen relative to the other two, that's known as *estrogen dominance*, and it can cause all sorts of problems.

Now, guys, don't stop reading once you hit the word "estrogen." Estrogen dominance primarily affects women, yes, but it can also affect you; in fact, the numbers of men with this problem are growing at an exponential rate. The ultimate effects are similar in both sexes, because unbalanced hormones spell trouble for your metabolism and your mood. And when estrogen dominance disrupts your thyroid, that is double trouble: You are likely putting on weight, dragging your feet every day, and losing your sex drive. In other rotten news, your hair is falling out, you're finding it harder to gain lean muscle mass, you crave carbs, and you might be suffering from depression.

Why are so many of us—male and female—struggling with estrogen dominance? One of the key reasons is *xenoestrogens,* toxins in our environment that behave like estrogens—a veritable wrecking ball to our glands and cells. For both men and women, estrogen is awesome in amounts the body can handle. But exposure to xenoestrogens throws the balance way off, not to mention causing DNA mutations that set us up for cancer. This link is discussed in a number of studies, including a 2006 article in the *Proceedings of the American Association for Cancer Research.* Research published in *Toxicologic Pathology* in 2009 also suggests a connection between xenoestrogens and breast cancer.

The problem is, xenoestrogens are everywhere. They are in everyday "conveniences" like our nonstick frying pans; in most plastics; in the pesticides found in non-organic produce; in water that's been exposed to industrial runoff; and in *parabens,* a common industrial chemical found in a wide variety of personal care products, including soaps, lotions, and shampoos. In fact, we are exposed to hundreds of xenoestrogens every single day: We eat them, we breathe them, and we put them on our skin—a serious problem when you consider that up to 65 percent of anything applied topically is absorbed by our bodies and can affect our weight and health. In 2016, researchers at the University of California–Berkeley asked 100 teenage girls to suspend using any of their normal cosmetics, lotions, and shampoos, relying only upon products free of common endocrine disruptors such as parabens and phthalates. In just three days, those girls' levels of hormone-disrupting chemicals dropped by 27 to 45 percent.

Xenoestrogens don't just disrupt our sex hormones, though. They also disrupt thyroid function.

First, estrogen dominance interferes with the conversion of T4 to T3. Remember, T4 is the storage form of thyroid hormone, while T3 is the active form. When your body can't activate that stored hormone, your whole metabolism slows down.

Estrogen also stimulates the production of thyroxine-binding globulin, which binds the thyroid hormone circulating in your bloodstream. Bound T4 can't convert into T3, and bound T3 can't enter your cells. So when you have too much estrogen in your system—and again, this applies to men, too—you don't have enough free T4 and free T3 to power your metabolism.

So what's our game plan? Use my tips in the next few chapters on choosing the right foods and exercise, and on reducing the effects of stress. I also want you to eat as "clean" as possible and to avoid parabens in your personal care products (check the labels!). Your thyroid will thank you for it, your metabolism will improve—and your scale will show the difference.

How to Avoid Endocrine Disruptors

A wonderful nonprofit organization called the Environmental Working Group (www.ewg.org) has a list of some of the products with the most endocrine disruptors—the hormone-altering chemicals that can undermine your thyroid and sabotage your metabolism. Here's a shortened version of their list and what you can do to avoid them. (To find out more about each saboteur or to learn about other endocrine disruptors, go to http://www.ewg.org/research/dirty-dozen-list-endocrine-disruptors.)

1. **BPA**: Used to line cans, coat receipts, and make some plastics. **Your plan**: Most canned foods contain BPA, so try to eat fresh food whenever possible (more nutrients!) or look for BPA-free cans. You might also want to avoid plastics whenever possible, especially BPA plastics.
2. **Phthalates**: Used in many types of plastics and personal-care products, often signaled by the term "fragrance." **Your plan**: Avoid plastic food containers and plastic wrap with the recycling label "3"; also read the labels carefully on personal-care products and avoid those with either "phthalates" or "fragrance" listed.

3. **Lead**: Found in old paint and drinking water.
   Your plan: Get rid of crumbling old paint—but carefully!—and install a water filter.
4. **Arsenic**: Found in drinking water and in brown rice.
   Your plan: Get a water filter, and limit your use of rice—especially brown rice and products that contain brown rice flour, such as protein powders and brown rice pasta.
5. **Mercury**: Found in large fish as the result of industrial pollution.
   Your plan: Avoid tuna and swordfish—stick to healthier fish.
6. **Perfluorinated chemicals (PFCs)**: Used to make nonstick cookware as well as stain-resistant and water-resistant coatings.
   Your plan: Avoid those products.

How to Nourish Your Thyroid

Besides being a demanding boss, your thyroid is kind of like a three-year-old picky eater. If it doesn't get the nutrients that keep it functioning in peak condition, it will do the equivalent of banging on the table and throwing the plate against the wall. So please, keep your thyroid happy by giving it the nutrients it needs.

The good news is that many of your "friendly foods"—the foods that work for you on The Metabolism Plan—contain precisely the nutrients that your thyroid needs. That's why this approach to eating is so effective at restoring thyroid balance.

Now, do you also need to take supplements? Well, I'm not a big fan of supplements taken regularly and long-term, although I think they are terrific as a short-term catalyst to optimal health. Ideally, though, I want you to get your nutrients from food, not shakes, bars, or pills. And you can! Time and time again, people come to me with a shopping bag of supplements and a laundry list of nutritional deficiencies, sure that they have to take the one to address the other. I ask them to stop taking everything and simply get their blood work done after just one month on The Metabolism Plan. Guess who no longer needs those supplements? How brilliant is that?

When you figure out which foods your body wants—your friendly foods—you will automatically be giving your thyroid (and the whole rest of your body) exactly what it needs. Suppose you're deficient in iodine—a common nutrient needed for optimal thyroid health. A food like cod or scallops is rich in iodine, so if it tests "friendly" for you, you can incorporate it into your diet. All of a sudden, you lose weight like a rock star and feel vibrant and glowing. Problem solved!

Or perhaps you are deficient in zinc, selenium, iron, and vitamin B12, all of which your thyroid also requires to function properly. Well, then, your body will love lamb, which is rich in those vitamins and minerals. And once again, problem solved!

So let's take a tour of your thyroid's key nutrients. Within 30 days you'll be eating all the foods you need to supply them.

Iodine

Your body needs iodine to make thyroid hormones. Sounds simple, right?

But life is often not so simple, and iodine is a case in point. Yes, studies have shown that diets that are too low in iodine can aggravate hypothyroidism. But so can diets that are too high in iodine. High intake of iodine might also increase the risk of Hashimoto's thyroiditis, an autoimmune condition in which your body is basically attacking its own thyroid gland.

I see this problem with a lot of my clients who keep taking iodine when they shouldn't. Has your doctor told you that you are deficient in iodine? If so, then yes, a little extra iodine—perhaps in the form of a supplement or some seaweed in your diet—will help to maintain proper thyroid function. Just be careful, because I have seen people who take iodine for too long go from being hypothyroid to becoming hyperthyroid.

How can you tell if you're in the hyperthyroid zone? Having your doctor order blood work is one great gauge. You can also do it yourself by taking your basal body temperature (BBT), a technique I teach you on page 45 and that you'll use throughout your 30 days and beyond to find out how various types of exercise affect your thyroid. Finally, you can check out the list of symptoms on page 30 to see whether you have the classic signs of hyperthyroidism: increased irritability, anxiety, sleeplessness, heart racing, muscle weakness, and trembling hands.

Meanwhile, if you are not iodine deficient, please! Save yourself some money, protect your little thyroid, and stop taking iodine supplements. Why spend money to make yourself sick? Your body will let you know if you need more iodine, and if it doesn't, then using sea salt and enjoying iodine-rich foods should supply you with all the iodine you need.

LOW-REACTIVE FOODS RICH IN IODINE:

Seaweed, cod, scallops, eggs, salmon sashimi, cranberries, and potatoes. (And that is why French fries can be good for both your thyroid and your weight loss! Mmmm.)

Selenium

After iodine, selenium is probably the most important mineral affecting thyroid function. T3 is your thyroid powerhouse, and your body needs selenium to convert T4 into T3. So many of your Metabolism Plan basics and least reactive foods make the selenium list!

LOW-REACTIVE FOODS RICH IN SELENIUM:

Chia seeds, sunflower seeds, flaxseeds, pumpkin seeds, shiitake mushrooms, chicken, beef, lamb, mussels, octopus, halibut, and bread. Although other experts often recommend Brazil nuts as a good source of selenium, I have found them to be highly reactive, probably because they absorb massive levels of radium, a naturally occurring source of radiation.

Zinc

Holy smoke, do I love zinc! The zinc-rich foods on The Metabolism Plan have really boosted my clients' ability to convert T4 into T3, with terrific results for metabolism, energy, and weight.

Men, here's a special benefit: Zinc is also great for prostate health. And for both sexes, zinc boosts immune function.

Now, don't rush right out and buy several bottles of zinc. The right amount of zinc is terrific, but too much can actually suppress thyroid function. Once again, let your body be your guide. Eating the friendly low-reactive foods you are naturally drawn to will eventually ensure that you're getting just the right amount of zinc for you.

LOW-REACTIVE FOODS RICH IN ZINC:

Pumpkin seeds, beef, lamb, chickpeas, shiitakes, chicken, oysters, and cocoa powder.

Iron

Iron deficiency is common among women—thanks again, monthly cycle! But you men aren't off the hook, because low iron levels are a risk for everyone as we age. Iron deficiency in turn affects our thyroid levels, because insufficient iron stores reduce our thyroid gland's ability to make hormone. And once again, you can eat your way to health.

LOW-REACTIVE FOODS RICH IN IRON:

Chicken, beef, lamb, haddock, lentils, pumpkin seeds, broccoli, liver, clams, mussels, salmon sashimi (but not cooked salmon—that's highly reactive!), apricots, almonds, basmati rice, raisins, green leafy vegetables, and potatoes.

Vitamin D

Vitamin D deficiency might increase your risk of autoimmune thyroid disease and is very common among people with thyroid cancer or thyroid nodules. Even if you are consuming enough vitamin D, you might not be *absorbing* it: If your small intestine isn't functioning up to par, it can't absorb all the vitamins you take in. And guess what? Impaired digestion is a hallmark of hypothyroidism. Talk about a vicious cycle! Luckily, The Metabolism Plan, a round of MSM, and a good-quality probiotic with no FOS (fructooligosaccharides) will help your thyroid and your digestion.

Stress can also sap your vitamin D levels by causing an increase of cortisol, a powerful stress hormone. Stress hormones are made from cholesterol, which your body needs to synthesize vitamin D from the sun. So when you are stressed, your body prioritizes the available cholesterol for stress hormones, with not enough left over to help with vitamin D production. A fabulous de-stressing supplement called SAM-e helps greatly on those days it seems like your world is exploding!

Happily, once you are on The Metabolism Plan, your vitamin D levels may bounce back very quickly, often within the month. Many of my clients have had this experience, and I'm betting you will get the same results!

LOW-REACTIVE, PLAN-FRIENDLY FOODS RICH IN VITAMIN D:

Wild whitefish, shiitake mushrooms, cheese, eggs, and organ meats such as liver, heart, and kidney. So break out the chopped liver or pâté and boost your vitamin D.

Vitamin B12

Almost half of hypothyroid patients are deficient in this crucial vitamin. And if you are vegan or vegetarian, your risk of deficiency is even greater.

As with vitamin D, your B12 deficiency might be caused by absorption issues. People with Hashimoto's, celiac, and other autoimmune diseases frequently have inflamed, damaged intestinal tracts, which prevents absorption of B12 and other nutrients. Intestinal issues and inflammation are common among overweight people as well. When you heal your gut on The Metabolism Plan, your absorption capacity will return.

LOW-REACTIVE, PLAN-FRIENDLY FOODS RICH IN B12:

Salmon sashimi, cod, lamb, scallops, beef, crab, cheese, and eggs.

Stress and Your Thyroid

When you're stressed, your body responds by producing more stress hormones, including the cortisol we've been talking so much about. In the right amounts, cortisol is amazing, fueling your energy, sharpening your mental focus, and motivating you to overcome any obstacle. In the wrong amounts, though, cortisol can make your life miserable—and it can disrupt thyroid function. As we just saw, cortisol production can monopolize resources that your body needs to make vitamin D. Since your thyroid needs vitamin D, this can be a problem.

Too much cortisol also disrupts the conversion of T4—the storage form of thyroid—into T3, the active form. It's as though, when you're stressed, your body starts to hunker down and conserve resources, slowing your metabolism and hanging on to every ounce of fat.

Stress relief is such an important topic that the whole next chapter is devoted to it. For now, let me just point out that stress disrupts thyroid function—and that the stress relief suggestions in Chapter 3 will be a huge help.

Getting the Right Exercise for Your Thyroid

Exercise is terrific! But is *any* type of exercise good? And if some is good, is more better?

The truth is a little more complex. There is a type and amount of exercise that's right for your body. When you get too much, too little, or the wrong type, your stress levels go up, your cortisol rises, and your thyroid suffers. You'll find out more about this fascinating process in Chapter 5. For now, just remember that the wrong type of exercise can disrupt thyroid function just as the right type of exercise can support it.

Sleep Your Way to Thyroid Health

I hope you got a chance to sleep in today! Not only is good sleep one of life's great pleasures; it is also one of the best possible ways to support your weight. Over years of working with a wide variety of clients, I have found that for every two hours of sleep you miss, you slow down your weight loss—guaranteed. That's a high price to pay for waking up early!

In a moment, I'm going to show you how to monitor your thyroid function by keeping track of your basal body temperature (BBT), a reading you can take with an ordinary thermometer. But here's a preview: When you've skimped on sleep, you can actually see your BBT drop—a clear measurement of thyroid disruption. And when your thyroid isn't working right, your whole metabolism slows down.

To make matters worse, lack of sleep starts to disrupt your entire hormonal system by kicking up a hunger hormone known as *ghrelin* and a brain chemical called endocannabinoid 2-AG (that resembles the same chemicals in cannabis), which combine to turn you into a snacking machine. It's hard to have a good weight-loss day when you feel ravenous! In the next chapter, you'll see that sleep issues also affect your adrenal glands and your cortisol levels, neither of which does any favors for your metabolism.

My Doctor Says My Thyroid Is Fine—But Is It?

Just about every conventional medical practitioner relies solely on the TSH test to see whether your thyroid is functioning optimally. But as you wise folks now know, TSH doesn't mean much if your body can't properly convert T4 to T3.

Moreover, the numbers for "normal" TSH are already skewed. The reference ranges for "normal" TSH levels were based on people who are not functioning optimally—people who came in because they didn't feel well. Even though those reference ranges have been challenged by the American Association for Clinical Endocrinologists as too wide, most doctors still use those problematic reference ranges. As a result, you could have a significant thyroid problem—but your test results will read "normal."

But on top of it—and this drives me crazy—the reference range is just that. A range. For example, suppose you are 5'6" and female. The range for your "normal weight" is 120 to 160. Let's say you have been 123 all your life and all of a sudden you step on the scale and you're 158. According to your doctor, that's still in the normal range. But it's not normal for you!

Your thyroid ranges work exactly the same way: Even if your numbers fall into the "normal" range, your thyroid function might not be normal for *you*. If you have been sailing along at a steady weight and then suddenly you start gaining, your TSH, free T4, or free T3 levels might have changed significantly while still remaining in the "normal" range. Your doctor says you are fine—but you're gaining weight and wondering why.

Another factor that can alter your thyroid status is whether you take birth control or are having hormone replacement therapy. Any type of extra estrogen stimulates the increase of the thyroid-binding proteins in your blood. So even if your thyroid is producing a "normal" amount of T4, too much of the T4 might be "bound"—tied up with the thyroid-binding proteins. And even if your T4 is converting properly to T3, too much of your T3 may also be bound. Since the bound thyroid hormone can't get into your cells, you effectively have low thyroid function, even though your lab results look okay.

Fortunately, the food and lifestyle tips in this book will help you support your thyroid, your powerhouse for best health and ideal weight. They'll help you overcome the effects of excess estrogen, and they'll also support the optimal conversion of T4 into T3. As a result, you might be able to avoid thyroid medication altogether, simply by giving your body what it needs. You'll feel better than ever before—and you'll be healthier, too.

How to Monitor Your Thyroid: Taking Your BBT

I'm all about empowering you with information and putting as many tools as possible into your tool belt. One of my favorite tools is a simple thermometer, which will give you an incredible amount of information every day—information that you can use immediately to boost your metabolism.

Your thermometer measures your basal body temperature (BBT), a direct indicator of how your thyroid is functioning. This test was developed by Dr. Broda Barnes, a great researcher into thyroid function who wrote books in the 1970s about how to use the BBT to accurately assess thyroid function. Dr. Barnes had noticed that many of his patients with major symptoms of thyroid dysfunction had blood work that was in a "normal" range. He wanted to find a better test of thyroid hormone levels, and with the BBT, he found one. His work is widely used by naturopathic physicians. (By the way, fertility specialists also use Dr. Barnes's work: They know that regardless of overall thyroid function, your BBT will generally rise during ovulation, and prior to your cycle starting.)

How to Take Your BBT

- Keep a digital thermometer by your bed at night.
- As soon as you wake up in the morning, place the thermometer in your armpit and hold it there for 2 minutes.
- Keep perfectly still: Any movement of the body can cause your temperature to rise.
- **Women:** Note that your BBT will rise when you are ovulating and five to seven days before your cycle starts, so it's important to keep

a full 30 days of data. During certain times of the month, some of my patients have a full 3-point jump in BBT!

- **Men:** You have hormonal fluctuations, too; they're just not as obvious as women's. Taking your BBT will give you a daily read on those ups and downs, allowing you to better understand your energy levels, mood, and ability to perform, both when working out and in everyday life. Feeling blah, weak, or irritable? Your BBT is most likely low. Feel like you can conquer the world? I bet you're operating in an optimal BBT zone: 97 to 97.3.

How Your BBT Helps You Develop Your Own Diet, Exercise, and Sleep Plan

When your thyroid gland is performing optimally, your BBT will be 97 to 97.3 degrees Fahrenheit. A functional zone can range from 96.5 to 96.9 degrees. If your temperature is consistently lower than 96.5 degrees, your thyroid is under-performing. If it's higher than 97.3 degrees, your thyroid may be over-performing.

I can't tell you how terrific this is as an instant check of your diet, exercise, sleep, and stress levels! Remember how I said your thyroid was a demanding boss? Well, it is, but it's also a very generous one. Please that boss, and you feel 100 percent:

- When a particular food works for you, your BBT will be in the optimal range the next morning. When a food doesn't work, your BBT will drop.
- When a particular type and intensity of exercise works for you, your BBT will be in the optimal range the next day. When you exercise too intensely, your BBT will drop.
- When you get the right amount of sleep, your BBT will hit the optimal zone the next morning. However, if your BBT goes down after six hours of sleep but achieves the optimal zone after seven or

eight hours, your body is talking to you loud and clear: Give me more sleep! If you listen, you'll get a big reward: enhanced weight loss.

Using the BBT protocol at my health center was instrumental when I first started focusing on thyroid issues. The traditional theory had the functional range at 97.2 to 97.8 degrees, but my team and I found something quite different. Remember, we work with people daily, monitoring their response to every kind of stimulus. Over thousands of patients, I've seen that the people I work with feel best at 97 to 97.3 degrees, a zone with great weight loss and digestion, vibrant energy and mood, and optimal health. When patients' BBT creeps up past 97.3, I start to see irritability, anxiety, sleeplessness, heart palpitations, hair loss, and sleep issues. That, my friends, is not optimal thyroid function; that's hyperthyroid issues!

Of course, you can have a high BBT and still feel hypothyroid. I usually see this with people suffering from high stress levels or adrenal burnout. The good news is that your 30 days on The Metabolism Plan are going to balance your hormones and endocrine system.

You'll learn exactly how to monitor your BBT in Part II as you develop your own personalized plan. Meanwhile, I promise you: This simple little tool is going to be one of your best friends when it comes to figuring out your exercise sweet spot. I want you feeling 110 percent not just once in a while but all the time. Taking your BBT will help get you there!

The Thyroid Promise

Every single day, you will be eating foods that help you reach all of your goals. You will also find the exercise that works for your body. Every day you will get leaner, stronger, and more energetic. Stop being a slave to the gym! I want you to get out there and enjoy this marvelous life you have created. And here's an additional bonus: Your thyroid medication might need to be cut by as much as 20 percent in as soon as three to five days!

How do you know when you are overmedicated? You'll be irritable and sleepless, with a racing heart or trembling hands because your thyroid has now started producing more hormone or your body is finally doing a good job of converting your T4 to T3. This is a terrific testament to how your body wants to heal, as soon as you give it what it needs. (As always, be sure to work with your doctor before altering or reducing your medication in any way.)

CHAPTER THREE

Stress and Your Metabolism

Okay, my dear friends, I'm going to tell you why stress makes you gain weight—regardless of how you eat and exercise. Stress isn't just a psychological state; it's a powerful biochemical response. And when you understand how it works, you'll know why it's a hugely important factor in your metabolism—and your weight. I can't change the stress in your life, but I can give you some awesome tools to mitigate its physiological effects on your body. Let's start by exploring where our stress response came from and why it works the way it does.

Many, many millennia ago, we humans were evolving into the complex biological creatures known as *Homo sapiens*. Life was rough and dangerous, and we didn't have much in the way of protection—no strong jaw, fangs, or claws, not even thick hides or super-speed to keep the predators at a distance.

And yet somehow, we managed to survive in some pretty fierce situations. What got us out of many a jam were survival skills—plus a biology that was geared to make the most of our physical, mental, and emotional resources.

So I want you to imagine you are sitting in a field, feeling pretty good, until suddenly you look up and see a tiger! Instantly you jump up and run faster than humanly possible, scrambling up a nearby tree or flinging yourself into a rushing river and swimming as hard as you can. And what enables you to perform these superhuman feats—this extra strength, this lightning-fast plan for escape? Stress hormones. Your trusty adrenal glands are participating in an elaborate biochemical cascade that begins in our brain and travels throughout our entire biology, commonly known as the "fight-or-flight" response, which enables you to outrun the tiger and live to see another day. And that's how the human race survived.

That superhuman effort takes a lot of energy. So when the stress reaction is working properly, you tap into fat as an energy source. Then, when the stressful event is over, you relax, the stress hormones leave your body, and your whole biochemistry shifts, replacing the stress response with the relaxation response, a.k.a. "rest and digest." You relax, digest your food, and eventually enjoy a deep, restful sleep that restores your exhausted body.

We're used to thinking of stress as bad—and it can be. But I would never wish for you a life without stress, because that would be the dullest life imaginable! Without the stress response, you'd never know that extra revving up when you rise to an occasion, prepare for an exciting challenge, or try to woo your one true love on the most important romantic date of your life. As you can see in the lists that follow, some types of stress are what give life its kick and its savor. Other types of stress are not so pleasant. Compare the two types:

Fun Stress
Learning something new
Falling in love
Riding a roller coaster
Working hard to achieve a cherished goal

Not-So-Fun Stress
Worries about money
Family problems—sickness, aging, arguments, etc.
Conflicts at work
Too much to do and not enough time to do it

Some types of stress start with your emotions or life situation. Others are physical:

Physical Stressors
Reactive foods
Too much exercise or the wrong type of exercise
Skimping on sleep
Missing meals

So here's your takeaway: As long as stress is replaced by relaxation, it won't affect your weight. But what if the stress never really goes away? What if you undergo too many stressful events too close together, or if the stress seems constant? *That's* the type of stress that causes you to gain weight. Even if you're eating and exercising in ways that are perfect for your body, stress that gathers and builds and doesn't go away can create a huge weight problem that is all the more painful because it seems so mysterious.

When the Stress Doesn't End...

For most of you reading this book, stress is primarily mental and emotional. Too many deadlines. A kid with learning disabilities, plus an aging parent, plus the threat of layoffs. Worries, demands, and challenges that never seem to let up, so that even during dinner, you're responding to work emails, and even after dinner, you're having an anxious phone call with tomorrow's babysitter, and even on the weekends, there's nothing but chores.

For most of us, that's twenty-first-century chronic stress. But back when our bodies were evolving, chronic stress meant something quite different: imminent danger, fire, floods, starvation. In such situations, your body has one job and one job only: to keep you alive. And body fat—both to keep you warm and to keep you from starving to death—is literally lifesaving. So when there's too much chronic stress, your body does something very special: It slows down your metabolism as far as it can. Your thyroid function drops as low as it can go. Your body stubbornly clings to every extra ounce of fat. And this state will continue just as long as the stress continues and maybe—just to be on the safe side—for some time after that.

If your primary concern today was to prevent starvation, you'd give thanks every night for this miraculous biological arrangement. But if your goal is to lose weight, you're fighting a tough battle, because as long as your body is struggling with chronic stress, it will strive to keep the fat on.

So what do you do? Probably what so many clients have told me they do: "cut calories" and skip meals to lose weight. I mean, that's what we were taught, right? If you want to lose weight, you need to cut calories. Maybe it's intermittent fasting or juicing. Maybe it's coffee drinks to curb hunger or maybe you just tough it out. However you cut calories, you have lost the belief that you can lose weight eating normally every day.

Well, that ends today! Weight loss does not mean punishment, and I want you to drop this punitive mind-set right now. Sure, starving yourself might give you temporary weight loss, but over the long term, skipping meals will actually cause you to gain weight because you're slowing the rate at which you burn the fuel that is your food.

By now you can probably guess why. When you miss a meal, your body thinks, "Starving! Starving!" and your entire metabolism grinds to the slowest possible pace, clinging to every extra ounce and lowering your metabolism. The body fat stays on, and you're feeling desperate. And that increased emotional stress just makes everything worse!

I know it seems counterintuitive, but it's absolutely true: Eating more will actually improve your ability to lose weight. So let's banish the 1,200-calorie mind-set. Start eating decent-sized regular meals right now and reassure your body that starvation is not a possibility.

Your Amazing Adrenals

Key to the whole stress experience is your adrenal glands, so let's take a look at them. In response to signals from your hypothalamus and pituitary—yes, the very same glands that direct your thyroid— your adrenal glands produce stress hormones.

Your brain perceives a potential threat.

It cues your hypothalamus.

Your hypothalamus releases biochemicals
that alert your pituitary.

Your pituitary releases biochemicals
that alert your adrenals.

Your adrenals release stress hormones that
flood your body and set off the stress
reaction described on page xv.

If your adrenals keep working overtime, cranking out too many stress hormones, you could end up with a condition known as adrenal burnout, in which your adrenals are producing the wrong levels of stress hormone at the wrong times of day. You might feel wired when it's time to sleep, exhausted when it's time to get up, or burned out all through the day. Excess stress creates other problems, also—for your metabolism, your weight, and your overall health.

Meet Your Stress Hormones

I want you to get to know your stress hormones, because they are crucial to a vital, energized, and inspired life. You have many different kinds of stress hormones, and their functions and operation often overlap. Here are a few key stress hormones, with a simplified description of each.

- **Adrenaline and noradrenaline (also known as epinephrine and norepinephrine)**: Ever hear of an adrenaline rush? These are the stress hormones it refers to. When you need to rev up for something quickly—a demanding deadline or an exciting first date—these hormones help power that state of being extra keyed up and alert.
- **Dopamine**: This stress hormone is what puts the thrill in a rollercoaster ride and the high in falling in love. Dopamine is your excitement hormone, fueling the anticipation you feel before a special vacation or your child's big award ceremony. It's also your uncertainty hormone, the one that comes into play when you gamble or take chances. Anxiously watching your favorite sports team, or taking physical risks (such as skiing or surfing) all rev up your dopamine.
- **Cortisol**: This is one of the most powerful stress hormones of all—and one of the most important factors in your health. Cortisol is the hormone that keeps you energized through the long slog of any demanding task, and when cortisol levels are low, you feel exhausted, unmotivated, or listless. Now, here's the good news: Once you get into a good relationship with your cortisol, you'll be able to achieve your dream body!

The Cortisol Connection

Cortisol can be your best friend or your worst enemy. In the right amounts, at the right times of day, cortisol is your fuel. Your cortisol levels should be highest in the morning; in fact, they are literally what give you the drive to get out of bed and start your day. This is known as your cortisol wakening response. All throughout the day, cortisol drops gradually until, by evening, it should be low enough for you to fall asleep. Then, in the morning, cortisol spikes upward to awaken you again, and the whole cycle starts over.

Now, we evolved to be flexible, and cortisol levels are part of that flexibility. So whenever you meet a challenge during the day, your cortisol levels spike to give you some extra energy. In a healthy body, a small challenge triggers a small cortisol spike; a big challenge triggers a big one. And with every challenge, you get that whole fight-or-flight stress-hormone cascade, because as far as your body is concerned, you just saw a scary tiger and you've got to be ready to move.

In a healthy body, each stress response is followed by a relaxation response, which allows your cortisol to fall back to wherever it was supposed to be (higher in the morning...lower in the afternoon...lowest at night). Your cortisol level spikes...and falls. You stress...and then relax. You keep rising to challenges...and then you stop feeling stressed and feel calm again. If that's the way your day goes, stress is not going to create weight gain.

But for all too many of us, that's not how the day goes. Instead, each new stressor stays with us and never really goes away. Stress accumulates, mounting every hour, until by the end of the day our cortisol levels are through the roof. In that state, even little things cause cortisol to spike much higher than it otherwise would, and to take much longer to fall back to normal.

To make matters worse, that high-stress moment at the end of the workday is when many of us choose to exercise. And since exercise is a stressor—you're challenging your body—that means your cortisol is spiking once again, just when it should be falling. Even worse, when your cortisol levels are chronically high—when the stress never really goes away—that, my friends, is when you gain weight and when your weight becomes nearly impossible to lose.

It makes sense, right? Your body doesn't know that you're stressing over deadlines and paying bills. It thinks you're being put through the incredible physical demands of famines and migrations through the desert. And so now your chronically heightened levels of cortisol lead to long-term fat storage, especially abdominal fat, which in the old days would have been used to fuel you in outrunning that tiger. To make matters worse, that abdominal fat contains higher levels of an enzyme that prods inactive cortisol to life. The more stress you have, the more cortisol you make—you've basically become a cortisol-producing machine! And through it all, your body is trying to do the right thing for a time of danger: slowing down your metabolism, conserving energy, and clinging to every ounce of body fat.

Kelly, Age 51

Since I started The Metabolism Plan, I lose weight eating cheese and chocolate, drinking wine, having pancakes for breakfast, enjoying appetizers when out with my friends, and eating the foods I love and enjoy! Thank you, thank you, thank you!

I have recommended The Metabolism Plan to so many people. And *every single person* who has tried it has expressed the same joy and amazement when the symptoms they suffer from improve and go away. My neighbor is no longer on reflux medicine, my friend's mother's joint pain went away, my friend's severe allergies cleared up significantly, and my neighbor's mother lost that 50-year-old bloat she thought she'd never get rid of. My only amazement now is that this approach is not being touted by every doctor as a miracle cure!

Cortisol and Your Thyroid

One of the ways your cortisol takes control of your metabolism is via your thyroid. Excess cortisol affects your thyroid in a number of ways:

- It decreases your production of TSH. As a result, your thyroid may not get the stimulation it needs.
- It prevents T4 (the storage hormone) from being converted to T3 (the active hormone).
- It promotes the conversion of T4 to reverse T3—the hormone that slows down T3 activity.

To make matters worse, when your cortisol is either too high or too low (which can happen after long periods of stress), it throws your blood sugar balance off. Your body reads that, too, as possible starvation—and once again, your thyroid slows down.

Cortisol, Thyroid, and Sex Hormones

Excess cortisol also disrupts your sex hormones: estrogen, progesterone, and testosterone. For both men and women, too much cortisol lowers your sex drive and your fertility. This makes sense if you picture, once again, humans in the wild, worrying about surviving extreme conditions and possible famine. Those are not the conditions under which a woman can easily support a pregnancy or breastfeed a newborn. And a physically threatened community can't easily take care of little children, either. When you're stressed, your body thinks it is in literal, immediate danger, and its top priority is staying alive, not creating new life.

Excess cortisol is one reason why young female athletes—whose bodies are stressed to the max—often don't get their periods on schedule, or why they sometimes stop menstruating. It's why adult women under stress might miss a period or struggle with irregular cycles and other hormonal difficulties. And it's why both men and women under stress might find themselves a lot less interested in sex. It's like your body is saying, "Whoa! Let's wait for a little more security before we make a baby!"

Here's something else that happens when cortisol stays too high for too long: Your liver starts to struggle. And since one of its jobs is to remove excess estrogen from your system, a poorly functioning liver means excess estrogen. Excess estrogen in turn leads to excess *thyroid-binding globulin,* a protein that binds to the thyroid hormone in your bloodstream and makes it inactive. So cortisol's effects on your estrogen levels also disrupt your thyroid. Once again, your metabolism slows down while your weight creeps up.

And guess what? Your body fat itself produces estrogen! So excess body fat gets you into a vicious cycle:

Excess body fat → excess estrogen → lowered thyroid
function → *more* extra body fat

At this point, you might feel like your whole body is set up to make you fat. Well, it sort of is—because we evolved in times where starvation was always a risk, so our bodies protect us by fighting starvation every way they can. The good news is that once you understand how your body works, you can reverse this cycle and give your body what it needs to be at a healthy weight.

So how do you keep excess cortisol from wreaking havoc on your metabolism? The solution is simple:

Make sure that any stress in your life is balanced by relaxation.

Believe me, I know that for many of us, that sounds about as easy as if I told you that the solution was to fly to Unicorn Mountain and bring home a rainbow. But don't worry—I've got some great and easy stress-relief suggestions that even the busiest, most stressed-out person can do. First, though, let's take a closer look at your body's age-old answer to the stress response: the relaxation response.

The Relaxation Response

Let's go back to seeing that tiger in the field. When your whole body mobilizes to fight or flee, it's governed by your *autonomic nervous system*. This is the system that supports all the responses you don't choose consciously: breathing, blood pressure, muscle tension, heart rate, and many others.

The autonomic nervous system has two halves: the sympathetic nervous system, which creates the stress response, and the parasympathetic nervous system, which creates the relaxation response. The key to a healthy metabolism is keeping those two halves in balance: every period of stress balanced by some relaxation.

Stress itself is not the problem. As we've seen, stress can be exciting and fun, and even when it's not, so what? You're tough—your body is built to handle challenges. The problem comes when stress isn't followed by relaxation—when the stress response occurs, over and over again, but the relaxation response does not kick in.

You've been there. You rush in the morning to get the kids out the door and pound the steering wheel in frustration as you navigate through a parking lot disguised as a freeway. You've got impossible deadlines before lunch and then you have to fight that same rush-hour traffic on the way home. You've got to get through dinner, help the kids with homework, and take care of a million other chores. By the time you go to bed, you're exhausted—but you're also wired, because the stress hormones have never really stopped coursing through your body. Then you wake up early to work off that muffin top. It's all stress and no relief...and that, my good friend, is not just bad for your spirits—it's absolutely terrible for your weight.

Now, for many of us, balancing stress with relaxation sounds like the most stressful challenge of all! Never fear—I've got lots of helpful suggestions, so read on.

Stress Relief: Your Key to Weight Loss

Here's the deal: You may not be able to make your worries and challenges magically disappear, but you *can* help your body recover from them. The key is awareness. If you know you've had a stressful day, figure out how to relieve that stress every single day. It doesn't have to take a lot of time—and it can make a world of difference. Here are some tools that will help you with stress relief.

SAM-e: Your Stress-Relief Supplement

SAM-e (s-adenosylmethionine) is an amazing supplement that has changed the lives of hundreds of thousands of people suffering from depression, stress, and stress-related weight gain. Although I'm not a big fan of using any supplement every single day on a regular basis, I do like supplements for helping your body short term or to support your transition out of depletion. And that's where SAM-e comes in— to help you shift out of stress.

In our office, Mondays are the most intense days, so everybody takes SAM-e. Tuesdays tend to be quieter, so we put the SAM-e back in the fridge. For my accountant clients, tax time is their stress-bomb season, so I tell them to start taking SAM-e on January 1st and not to stop until April 15th. You get the idea: Use SAM-e whenever you need to bring your stress down to manageable levels.

What if stress hits you out of the blue? Take SAM-e right away: You'll feel calm almost immediately. Now little things won't drive you crazy, and your stress will *stay* manageable. Better yet, SAM-e will keep your body from clinging to belly fat because it keeps you out of the "danger zone," in which everything that happens just makes you feel more and more and more stressed.

Meditation

Did you know that meditating for even a few minutes a day can decrease the size of your *amygdala,* the part of your brain that is responsible for autonomic responses associated with fear and anxiety? Meditation can also increase the size of your *prefrontal cortex,* the part of your brain associated with reasoning and logic. Look, I'm like you, and my day is packed to the gills, but even I can find five minutes to meditate. Some of my favorite quick, guided meditations are listed in the Resources.

You can also incorporate "mindfulness meditation" into your normal day. Simply step away from your desk for five minutes, breathe deeply, find something to focus on—a tree, the sky, a photograph or painting—and let yourself be in the moment. I like to set the timer on my phone to a peaceful song, so I can give myself over to relaxation until it goes off.

I am going to say this loud and clear: One of the most effective ways to decrease stress and enhance weight loss is meditation. I promise you, it's easier than you think!

Inspirational Books or Sayings

Finding words that inspire you can shift your body from stress mode into the relaxation response, so start collecting awesome quotes and books to use whenever you need a stress-relief break. Here is one of my favorite quotes ever, from my friend Ingrid Marcroft, a wonderful yogini and the owner of Upper West Side Yoga and Wellness in New York City:

> *Befriend your body. Your body is unique and has stories like none other in the world. It is always changing. While walking down the street, while sitting or lying down, be amazed by what your body can do instead of what it can't do. Fall in love with your body.*

Cranking Up the Tunes

Remember your favorite songs from when you were young? Break them out and have an all-out jam. Move your body and revel in memories. Remember, music can evoke joy like few other things, so use singing, dancing, and listening to lower your cortisol.

Caring for Others

Whether it's adopting a pet, volunteering at a soup kitchen, or spending an hour a week to help a child learn how to read, helping others makes us feel *good*. Time crunched? Just look through your closet and realize that all those clothes you saved for your heavy days will be gone soon. You can donate those and help others in need.

Sleep: When Your Body Restores

Sleep is literally your shift out of the stress response to the relaxation response—from high alert to letting down your guard. That's why sleep is the ultimate way to balance your sympathetic and your parasympathetic nervous systems, and why you need deep, restful, and sufficient sleep every night.

Sleep is also essential for optimal thyroid function and increasing human growth hormone (HGH) levels. Both HGH and your thyroid will help reverse the aging process and get you your dream body. Sleep also helps to regulate two hormones that are essential for weight loss: leptin and ghrelin. Leptin is the hormone that says, "You're full, put down the fork." Ghrelin is the hormone that says, "You're starving, let's go back for a third helping." Lack of sleep causes leptin to fall and ghrelin to rise, so you feel like you're starving all day. Over-exercise pushes leptin levels down even further, so if your workout is too intense, you will also have a harder time feeling full. There should be some major light bulbs going off right now!

Need some help getting good sleep? Here are my favorite natural sleep aids.

Lemon Balm: Terrific for Both Stress and Sleep!

One of my favorite herbs is lemon balm, a.k.a. *Melissa officinalis*. This soothing, de-stressing herb is a member of the mint family and has been cultivated in Europe for thousands of years.

Like all members of the mint family, lemon balm supports digestion. Most of your serotonin—a feel-good hormone that fights depression and supports sleep—is produced in your gut. So it make sense that when you support digestion, you also support better mood and calm a frazzled nervous system. Over the past 20 years, research confirms what we have seen with our own Metabolism Planners: Lemon balm is incredibly effective at establishing a sense of peace in situations of high anxiety and stress. Lemon balm also improves quality of sleep, reducing restlessness and insomnia.

I usually have my clients take 500 mg of the standardized extract. Most of our clients who take lemon balm don't notice excess drowsiness but only a lovely sense of calm. If you do feel sleepy, try taking it only at night.

Please use lemon balm only on an as-needed basis. If you are experiencing a long period of high anxiety, you might want to alternate: one month of lemon balm and one month of hops (read on!).

Hops

Most of us know hops as the ingredient in beer that gives it its bitter, malty flavor. But the benefits of hops aren't limited to breweries: They've been used by herbalists for thousands of years, and now many of my clients are seeing benefits as well.

Hops have long been studied for use in anxiety, sleep disorders, and hormonal issues. They are an amazing sleep aid with a very potent calming effect. Unlike lemon balm, which tends not to have a sedative effect (just a calming one), hops is more of a sedative, so please save it for nighttime only.

Penny, Age 46

In a short few months, my weight ballooned by over 20 pounds. I had absolutely no energy and was edgy, anxious, and not thinking clearly. I was not me. I am not crazy, yet doctor after doctor thought I was. My gynecologist said that I would never again feel the way I did when I was 40. Really? I was only 46. Test after test, only to be told that this was my "new normal." I was sick and tired of being sick and tired.

So I contacted Lyn-Genet, and she changed my life. Now I have energy. I have clear thoughts. I am no longer edgy. I have lost 13 pounds without dieting or counting calories. I know my body and now I have the tools to interpret what my body is telling me. I thought that I was already a healthy eater—how on earth did I miss an apparent lifelong sensitivity to cow's dairy? My lifelong stomachache, which I've had since childhood, disappeared after I began working with Lyn-Genet's very talented, caring staff.

My husband is thrilled to have his happy, energetic wife back. He enjoys several of my new recipes and often cooks dinner for us when I am working late. Being on The Metabolism Plan is a commitment to my health, but it is not weird or full of rules. I eat real food. I even eat out frequently due to the demands of my job. The Metabolism Plan is exactly that—a plan for feeling the best that I can. Thank you for changing my life.

CHAPTER FOUR

The "Healthy Eating" Trap

I'm sure you've heard the old saying, "Knowledge is power"? That's my motto, and it's how I want you to operate. The Metabolism Plan is based on you gathering information about every aspect of your diet—which foods and even which restaurants work for you. This isn't some diet regimen that you mindlessly follow, stuck with the same "no's" forever. This is your opportunity to create your very own personalized diet and exercise plan, fine-tuned to your body, changing as your body changes, so that you are always in peak physical, mental, and emotional condition.

Your body speaks to you in a dozen different ways, every day, all the time. That twinge in your left knee? That's your body saying, "Inflammation! Eggplant is not for us." That foggy feeling when you hit four o'clock and want to fall asleep at your desk? That's your body saying, "Too much animal protein at lunch!" That exhausted feeling post-workout? That's your body saying, "Boot camp doesn't work—*please* switch to something gentler!"

The Metabolism Plan is based on you listening to your body. Every morning you will take your temperature, and every day you will weigh yourself. (More about that in a minute, but you'll learn to love the scale, I promise!) Those readings will show you exactly how

your body feels about what you're giving it to eat and how you're asking it to exercise.

Like anything else, understanding your body takes practice, but in
this case it's just relearning a language you used to speak. Throughout your first 30 days on The Metabolism Plan, you'll get much better
at interpreting what your body is saying and figuring out the foods
that are right for you. So many people have told me that they forgot
what it's like to have pain-free days, days where they weren't bloated,
constipated, and achy. They thought that feeling bad was now their
new norm. Well, pretty soon, feeling *good* will be your new norm—
and any bad feeling will be a clear message that empowers you to
take effective action.

You are the one who will decide which foods you can eat and
which you should avoid for now. You won't have to guess or wonder why those numbers on the scale seem so random. You will be
testing—getting your own personal data on your own biochemistry
and developing a bio-individual diet.

This is just as true for exercise as for food, by the way. As you will
see in Chapter 5, some of you can benefit from CrossFit, while others
should stick to swimming or rock climbing or yoga. Both the food and
the exercise your body loves will probably change over the years, and
when you understand how your body works, you'll be able to keep
changing your diet and your workout regimen to fit your body.

There Is No Such Thing as Healthy—Only What's Healthy *for You*

So here's what you're going to do. After a three-day cleanse in which
you'll rest up and allow your body to heal, you're going to test food on
even-numbered days and exercise on odd-numbered days. By "test,"
I mean that you'll try out either a new food or a new form of exercise. Every morning, you'll take your BBT to see how your thyroid
is reacting, and you'll weigh yourself to see whether you've had an
inflammatory reaction to anything you did the day before. (Remember, inflammation causes your body to gain weight immediately.)

This is going to be great, because you will know for sure whether a food or exercise is right *for you*. If it is, stick with it. If not, drop it. By the end of 30 days, you will have amassed a long list of friendly foods that you know will keep you at a healthy weight, and friendly exercise that you know is right for your body. You'll have figured out which foods to stay away from—at least right now. (You can always retest them, and as we'll see later on, you *should* keep retesting.) You'll know which exercises stress you out and cause you to gain weight. Armed with this knowledge, you'll be eating and exercising exactly the way your body needs—and the payoff is your dream body.

Here's the basic science:

- The foods that make you gain weight and provoke your symptoms are the ones that trigger inflammation.
- Everybody's body chemistry is different—a unique response to your history, genetics, environment, and lifestyle. Therefore, each of us has a different list of foods that trigger inflammation.
- To learn which foods are most likely to trigger inflammation ("reactive foods"), check out the chart on page 14—but remember, these are the numbers for most people. Your own responses might well be different, which is why you're going to test every single food. Because I want to lay the odds in your favor, you'll start with the foods that are least reactive for most people, so you can quickly put together a list of friendly foods that will become your mainstays.
- No matter how healthy a food is supposed to be, it might be reactive *for you*. If so, you'll immediately gain weight, develop symptoms, or both.
- The amount of weight you gain tells you just how reactive a particular food is for your chemistry. If you gain only 0.1 pound, that food is not the worst thing in the world and you can probably enjoy it every so often. If you gain 2 pounds, that's a highly reactive food for you, so avoid it now and retest in a year or so.

Here's one last key point, and it might be my most important point ever:

A lot of so-called healthy foods are actually reactive for a lot of people, especially as we age.

It's distressing to know that your weight has been going up from so-called healthy foods like tofu or quinoa. And maybe for *some* people these foods *are* healthy. For many of us, however, "healthy" foods like hard-boiled eggs, bananas, and Greek yogurt are the gateway to inflammation, premature aging, digestive disorders, and chronic pain.

The good news is, you will finally learn exactly what causes you to gain weight and what causes you to lose it. It all starts with inflammation, so let's take a closer look.

The Inflammation Factor

Inflammation is your body's response to an infection or injury. When you get a cold, inflammation helps your body to fight off the rhinovirus that provoked it. If you sprain your ankle, inflammation helps your body to repair the injury and return to health.

As inflammation does its healing work, it brings with it a range of effects that are not always so pleasant: *heat, redness, swelling,* and *pain.* When you get a cold, for example, you often feel feverish (*heat*). Your nose turns red or maybe your whole body is flushed (*redness*). Your nasal passages swell (*swelling*). You might feel achy all over (*pain*). These are the side effects of your immune system working to heal your body.

Likewise, with a sprained ankle, you can feel the flesh around your ankle get warm. Your ankle turns red and swells up. It hurts. These are the side effects of immune-system chemicals as they heal and repair the injury. Inflammation can be a good thing—but its side effects are not always so great.

When inflammation subsides after the threat is over, its side effects go away. Your cold is over. Your sprain is healed. And look! The redness, swelling, heat, and pain are gone, too. That's what's known as *acute* inflammation—a short-term response that quickly goes away.

But what if inflammation becomes *chronic,* as when your immune system is continually reacting to a set of triggers that never really go away? Then you've got problems, because now those side effects become permanent and turn into a wide variety of symptoms:

- Arthritis
- Brain fog
- Chronic pain
- Digestive issues such as constipation or IBS
- Fatigue
- Headache, migraine
- Hormonal imbalance
- Loss of sex drive
- Mood issues such as anxiety, depression, and irritability
- Skin conditions such as eczema and psoriasis
- Weight gain.

So how does inflammation become chronic? What kinds of triggers can keep provoking inflammation again and again and again—until, finally, it and its symptoms take up permanent residence in your body?

Two key triggers are reactive foods and the wrong kinds of exercise. When you keep eating foods your body can't tolerate, or exercising in a way that doesn't suit you, your body responds with inflammation, which, over time, becomes chronic. The weight comes on and stays on, your symptoms become "the new normal," and you begin to feel as though your body were the enemy. It's not—you just need to stop provoking that chronic inflammation.

Inflammation and Your Gut

Your gut is a huge factor in chronic inflammation. If your digestive tract is in poor shape—which can happen due to stress, lack of sleep, problematic food choices, and a host of other reasons—the tight junctions in your small intestine loosen up, allowing partially digested bits of food to leak through. This is known as *intestinal permeability* or *leaky gut*. Since most of your immune system is located just on the other side of your intestinal wall, it gets first look at this undigested food, and it does not like what it sees. Because your immune system knows only how to recognize the pure nutrients extracted from *fully* digested foods, all that partially digested food appears to be an invader.

When your immune system is under attack, it mobilizes its defenses: antibodies that will sound the alert anytime an invader appears. So when you put some milk in your coffee or take a bite out of your breakfast omelet, your immune system says, "I remember that partially digested milk! I remember that partially digested egg! Attack! Attack!" Milk, eggs, or whatever other food your immune system has tagged with antibodies is now considered armed and dangerous, and your immune system will respond with inflammation every time that food appears.

That's how you get low-grade chronic inflammation—you trigger it every time you eat a food that your immune system has learned to mistrust. You gain weight and start to experience health issues. And you start to think your body is the enemy when it's only doing its best to protect you.

The *really* bad news is that chronic inflammation also sets you up for some serious illness down the road. Heart disease, diabetes, autoimmune conditions, and even cancer can result. For both your weight *and* your health, you want to reduce chronic inflammation as far as possible.

To make matters worse, getting older means that your digestive system tends to lose a bit of resilience. You can have fewer digestive enzymes, and stomach acid and even saliva can decrease. You might have further compounded gut dysfunction by years of stress, missed sleep, and problematic food choices. Over time, as your gut function deteriorates, stress keeps building, and your inflammation mounts, you create a kind of perfect storm.

In my previous book, I talked about Jerry, a 25-year-old who had a mild sensitivity to wheat and tomato sauce. But he was young and his digestion was still operating at near-peak levels, so he never really noticed the beginning of digestive issues.

After ten years of enjoying pizza three nights a week, though, his poor immune system had had enough. And because he had lost some digestive enzymes, his body was having more trouble digesting these reactive foods. He had also lost some resilience in his *microbiome,* the community of gut flora that you need in order to digest your food, support your immune system, and keep your brain in peak condition. Stress, lack of sleep, disrupted thyroid function, and a whole host of other factors had put Jerry's immune system through a lot of changes, so that what had once appeared to his immune system as a little threat now began to look like a big one. Instead of saying, "Oh, pizza, well, I guess I can handle it," his immune system began to say, "Pizza, again? It's too much! Send out the killer chemicals! Send out the inflammation! Let's burn out this threat!"

In other words, when you don't recognize that foods are triggering inflammation, you keep eating them—and your inflammation skyrockets. You gain a pound or two overnight. And the inflammatory symptoms on page 69 start spinning out of control.

Once you get into an inflammatory downward spiral, things tend to get even worse. In your mid-20s, you had a mild reaction to tomatoes and pizza dough. In your mid-30s, your reaction gets more severe, plus you're also starting to react to eggplant, salmon, and walnuts. By the time you turn 40, your immune system is panicking when you introduce cauliflower and strawberries, and it's not too thrilled with arugula, raspberries, or milk. Your seemingly healthy diet is packing on the pounds and triggering the symptoms. You feel like the only way you can lose weight is to eliminate any food that's fun. Or else you just plain give up.

Now, here's the good news: As soon as you reverse this vicious cycle, a whole lot of terrific things begin to happen.

- You strengthen digestion so that foods that used to be reactive stop being a problem.
- You lose weight and maintain your ideal weight eating normal foods that you love.
- By supporting optimal digestion, you also support optimal mood.
- Your overall health improves.

The Gluten Go-Round

"Lyn-Genet, can I have gluten?"

I get asked this all the time, and I have a simple answer: "Let's test it." Only 20 percent of people tend to react negatively to wheat, so there's a good chance it may work for you now or in the future.

Of course, if you have celiac disease, that's another story. Celiac disease is an autoimmune condition in which gluten erodes your *villi*, the delicate projections from your intestinal wall. This interferes with digestion and undermines your ability to absorb nutrients from the food you eat. So if you have celiac disease, you must 100 percent avoid gluten. End of story.

Now, what about the rest of us? Some people seem to have no trouble digesting gluten—but have been told by nutritionists that gluten should be avoided. Others do seem to be gluten sensitive, developing weight gain and other symptoms when they consume gluten.

To some extent, that adverse reaction has to do with age. It's possible that you could once tolerate gluten and now you can't because you were overdosing on gluten through daily pasta and bagels. However, The Metabolism Plan radically reduces your levels of inflammation, so within a few weeks or months, you might actually be able to have gluten a few times a week.

My son is a great example. He had a mild wheat allergy, so I had him avoid all wheat for a year. Now his digestion has healed and he can enjoy bread and homemade pizza made with Caputo's flour from Italy, which you can order on Amazon.

So here's what we're going to do. We're going to test gluten and see how you react to it. If gluten passes your body's test, no problem—enjoy it in moderation (because you want to enjoy just about everything in moderation; overdoing a food is one of the quickest ways to develop a reaction to it). If gluten causes you to gain weight and feel lousy, avoid it—and maybe retest it in six months or a year.

I don't want to demonize gluten, especially because so many of the gluten-free alternatives are made with corn, tapioca starch, and potato starch, and these ingredients can be even more inflammatory than gluten. As with every other food, ask your body. You'll always get the best possible answer.

Salt Is a Four-Letter Word

Do you know which food is the sneakiest saboteur? S-A-L-T, which finds its way into processed foods, packaged foods, and restaurant foods to a truly disturbing extent.

Now, don't get me wrong: We need *some* sodium, which is a vital electrolyte that helps to regulate bodily fluids, cellular activity, and nervous function. The amount of sodium that most of us consume, however, is way over the top. Adding insult to injury, excess sodium also provokes sugar cravings. Plus, excess iodized salt is a risk factor for thyroid disease.

I find that most people do best with 1,500 to 2,500 mg of sodium per day. You'll be on the higher end if you are athletic, especially in times of heat and high humidity, because you'll excrete more sodium through your sweat.

It's hard to avoid salt if you don't know where it lurks, so here's a provocative question: Which type of packaged food is the biggest source of sodium in most people's diet? The answer might surprise you: *bread.*

There are others that might surprise you, too—for instance, chicken. Wait a minute—*chicken*? Yes, because chicken is often highly salted when you buy it prepared or as kosher chicken. Even that diet staple, a poached chicken breast, was most likely marinating in chicken broth rich in sodium *and* MSG, causing seemingly inexplicable weight gain.

And that quick and easy low-cal soup? I just looked at a can of virtuous, "diet-friendly" organic lentil soup. A single serving had only 130 calories, but 980 mg of sodium! And I don't know about you, but those servings are usually pretty darn small!

So please, watch out for the hidden salt and let's go easy on the saltshakers so your palate can open up to other flavors. Reducing salt is like turning down the volume on a blasting radio and suddenly hearing the sounds of nature that you had been missing all this time. Without an overload of salt, your flavor vocabulary will expand, and so will the pleasure you take in food. Plus many of the spices and seasonings you can use instead of salt have health benefits: They are often antibacterial and antimicrobial, and they can even help to lower cholesterol and balance blood sugar.

Forget About Calories—Focus on Chemistry

If I followed the calorie charts for my height, I'd be living on 1,100 calories a day. Instead, I consume more than 2,000, and I'm lean and energized. So let's lose that calorie myth and focus on nutrition and what makes you feel good. A hundred calories of almonds would obviously react differently than a hundred calories of donuts, right?

When you do your three-day cleanse right at the beginning of the Plan, you'll consume roughly 2,000 calories if you're a woman and 2,800 if you're a man—and you'll probably lose at least 5 pounds. Your goal is to identify what causes *inflammation.* Reduce the inflammation, and the weight will melt away.

Inflammation and food reactions are so highly individual, it's mind-boggling—but at this point, hopefully, this is making a lot of sense to you. For example, two common dietary triggers are beans and bell peppers, as I know all too well. If I take even a bite of hummus or eat a sliver of pepper, my sinuses clog and I gain a pound. But I have clients blithely eating both, as happy as can be.

Recently I was in Houston seeing clients, and I had dinner with Jackie, one of my staff. As you can imagine, when people go out with me they are on their "best behavior," so Jackie ordered all of her friendly foods and we chose a nice bottle of wine. I heard a small sigh and asked her what was wrong. She looked up at me and said two words: "Fried calamari."

"C'mon, Jackie, let's order some," I said. "It will be fun!" Her eyes opened wide in surprise, but she wasn't complaining. It was a great meal, full of laughs, and the next morning I received a delighted email: Jackie was down a pound, and now she had a new dish and a new restaurant to put on her friendly list!

Don't Fear Your Cravings—and Don't Worry About "Falling Off the Wagon"

"Lyn-Genet, I just find myself craving sugar—and I know it's bad for me. How do I make the cravings go away?"

"For me, it's starches. Potatoes, pasta, beans, anything starchy—I just want more and more and *more*."

One of the most wonderful things about discovering what works for your chemistry is the way it makes all your cravings go away. Many of my clients tell me they struggle with uncontrollable cravings, only to discover, after the cleanse, that they are totally craving-free. What's going on?

When you have inflammation in your digestive tract, it can cause a rise in *ghrelin*, the hormone that regulates hunger. Ghrelin provokes you to think you're hungry when you really don't need any more food. Because hunger is meant to be a warning sign of starvation—that is, low blood sugar—excess ghrelin often causes you to crave foods that will quickly drive your blood sugar up: sugars and starches.

Ghrelin levels also rise in response to low levels of thyroid hormone, as well as lack of sleep. This makes sense, because we know that when your body is under stress—when it believes that it's in danger of starving to death or dying of the cold—your thyroid production slows way down, trying to conserve energy. At the same time, you feel hungrier, which is your body's way of trying to fatten you up. If you were trekking across the tundra or facing a long, cold winter, it would be useful to feel hungry as often as possible, so that you'd be ready to take advantage of any food source that came into your reach. So please, don't be mad at your body—it's only trying to save your life!

Here's one more factor that creates cravings. Reactive foods create yeast, a type of intestinal fungus. Yeast just *loves* sugar, so when your intestinal yeast population starts to multiply in response to a reactive food, it creates in you intense cravings for sweets and starches to a sometimes overwhelming extent.

To make matters worse, excess exercise depresses your levels of leptin, the hormone that lets you know when you are full. Are you starting to see how right now you aren't set up to win? I'm going to help you change all of that, and pronto!

So I want you to say to yourself, *It's not me. I'm not out of control. These cravings have just been my natural reaction to eating foods that were reactive for me.* Maybe those monster workouts were causing monster cravings by suppressing leptin. Or maybe you are reactive to grilled salmon. But now that you understand the biology of your hunger and your appetite, you don't have to worry that your cravings are about lack of willpower. They absolutely are not. I've worked with people who weighed 400 pounds, and I promise you, willpower wasn't the issue: Biology was. Just knowing that should help you give yourself a break. Plus you will support your thyroid function, get the right exercise, and eat the right foods, so that neither thyroid nor inflammation will be disrupting your metabolism.

By the way, contrary to what you may have heard, small amounts of sugar are *not* the problem either. Just as likely, that turkey burger you were reactive to was what turned you into a cookie-eating fiend! Or asparagus, or bell peppers, or whatever your trigger foods are. As we've seen, *inflammation* is the real problem. So please don't demonize any foods. Instead, learn how to analyze what does and doesn't work for your body.

How The Metabolism Plan Works

- **The Cleanse (Days 1 to 3):** You'll start with a three-day food-based cleanse—three full meals plus a snack each day, using the foods that my research has found to be least reactive. This will bring your inflammation levels down quickly while giving your body a break from heavy digestion, allowing it to repair and restore. You're likely to lose about 5 pounds if you're a woman, and 7 to 10 pounds if you're a man—but don't worry if it's more or less. Weight loss is coming, soon enough!

- **Laying the Groundwork (Days 4 to 10):** After the cleanse, you begin to build a solid foundation of foods that are friendly to your body. In this phase, most of the foods and types of exercise are likely to agree with you, so much so that people like to call this the honeymoon phase.

  - On even-numbered days, you'll test a new food. That is, you will include a new food in one of your meals and then weigh yourself the next day. If your weight drops, the food is friendly. If your weight goes up, the food is inflammatory for you. If your weight stays the same, the food is mildly reactive and will be cut for now, since it will interfere with your testing. After your 30 days, please feel free to enjoy this food on days you don't test. So if one of your favorite foods is mildly reactive, don't despair—you can still have it every so often, as long as you follow it with a low-inflammatory day. It's only when you have inflammatory day after inflammatory day that you start to see health and weight issues. You'll continue testing until you have 40 or 50 friendly foods that you can rotate to create a healthy food plan *for you.*

- On odd-numbered days, you'll test a new type of exercise. Again, the next day you will weigh yourself and take your BBT. These measurements will let you know whether the exercise is friendly to your body or provokes weight stabilization or weight gain. Just as with foods, you'll eventually build a battery of exercise types and amounts that will work for you.

- **Step It Up (Days 11 to 20):** Now you'll be testing more reactive foods on your even-numbered days, and exercise that's 20 percent more intense on your odd-numbered days. You'll be losing weight most of the time as you learn more about what types of food and exercise are right for your body.

- **Fine-Tuning (Days 21 to 30):** In this phase, *you* pick which foods and exercise you want to test, continuing to learn what does and doesn't work for you.

The goal, as you can see, is to make this not *my* plan, but *your* plan. Sounds good, yes? The Metabolism Plan is designed for you to lose about half a pound each day until you reach your set weight and feel terrific. If you lose less weight than that, if you gain weight, or if you have any negative response whatsoever, it's for one of the following four reasons:

- You didn't drink enough water, or you drank water after dinner (see page 135).
- You've had too much sodium (see page 73).
- You've eaten a food that is reactive for you.
- You exercised too much, or did the wrong type of exercise.

Every day, you'll be hopping on the scale and taking your temperature, so you'll have these objective measurements to tell you whether a food is reactive. If your BBT dips or your weight goes up, that food isn't working for you. You might also develop a symptom—a headache, a drop in energy, a rush of anxiety, or perhaps even a stronger reaction. Your body has had a chance to heal during your three-day cleanse; it got used to not being assaulted by inflammatory foods. So when you introduce a trigger food that provokes an inflammatory reaction, you sometimes get a super-intense reaction as your body jumps in surprise. "*What?* I thought we were done with that, and now you're bringing it back again. *Noooo!!!!*"

Whether your response is weight gain, an intense physiological response, or both, you'll know that your body *really* doesn't like this food, or at least, not right now. Honestly, this is good news: Now you know to stop eating that food. Even better, you know that *this* is part of the reason your weight and health have been thrown off track. Cut this food out of your life—at least for now—and watch your weight drop and your health bounce back.

A food reaction can last 72 hours. The good news is that once you cut that food out, have your friendly foods the next day, and take a probiotic (to restore gastrointestinal balance), you should rapidly heal, losing any weight you gained as a reaction. And that's why we alternate: We test foods only every other day, and the same with exercise. We want to give your body a chance to get back to baseline.

What if you feel like you need an extra day or two when you have a severe reaction (like, say, 2 or more pounds of weight gain)? It's okay: Just don't test the food that was scheduled for that day; eat only friendly foods that you know will work for you. You can always come back to that day and test later.

Why Not Just Use the ALCAT Test to Find Your Food Sensitivities?

People often ask me about taking the Antigen Leukocyte Antibody Test, better known as ALCAT, a common food allergy test. I always tell them that both ALCAT and the other food sensitivity tests available can be confusing because so many variables can affect your testing. Here are just a few:

1. During times of seasonal allergies, or if you're around pets to which you are allergic, you're in a heightened histamine state. That means you will test allergic to many more foods than you otherwise would.
2. Times of hormonal fluctuations may influence how you do with your food tests. So if you start to notice you are testing reactive to all of your foods right before your cycle starts, stay with your friendly foods and friendly days. But you can still keep exercising. Luckily your body seems to do better with more exercise right before your cycle starts!
3. Heightened levels of cortisol will make you test sensitive to more foods. So if you have a fight with your spouse, or have a deadline at work, your blood work might be very inaccurate.
4. The "rotate or react" principle also affects your testing. If you ate spinach five days in a row before your test, guess who is going to test as allergic to spinach? This is one I see quite often!
5. You can even get different results if you take your blood test in the morning or in the afternoon!

Jacqueline, Age 45

I've paid tons of money for the ALCAT for my 18-year-old daughter, who has ankylosing spondylitis. We tested her three different times, and she never got results by avoiding the foods it said she reacted to.

I told my daughter about The Metabolism Plan and explained the commitment it would take to do it. I offered to do it with her and we were buying vegetables I'd never heard of and using spices I'd never used before! It was an adjustment, but when you see the scale going down and your energy levels going up, there's no stopping you.

Usually, on scale of 1 to 10, her pain level was at an 8, including nighttime. She had not been able to find relief standing, sitting, or lying down. On Day 5, I asked whether her pain was any better and she smiled at me and said, "I'm about a 4 now." I was so happy for her, I almost cried.

One day we were in a rush to get to my son's wrestling tournament, so we literally ran from the parking area. Suddenly my daughter shouted, "Mom, look at me, I'm running and it doesn't hurt!" We both laughed so hard. It was *awesome*, and a memory I will never forget. Thank you so much for giving that to me and my daughter.

To sum it up, the ALCAT was way off. The Metabolism Plan was dead-on. I'm so grateful we were able to cancel her appointment with a rheumatoid arthritis specialist. She feels so blessed to have learned the proper way to eat at such a young age. Lyn-Genet, you have our eternal thanks!

Listen to Your Body

One of the saddest things I see in my practice—and I see it all the time!—is people who think their bodies have turned against them. People are always telling me, "I gain weight if I just *look* at food."

It's easy to understand why you feel this way. You think your body has been betraying you. But now you know, whenever you gain weight in response to a healthy stimulus like food or exercise, that's your body saying, "Please stop. This doesn't work for us."

If you think about it for a minute, that's pretty amazing. All you have to do is listen to your body and it will guide you to the diet and exercise that will keep you at an ideal weight, feeling 110 percent and loving life.

CHAPTER FIVE

Exercise

Finding Your Balance

What if I told you that you could have a million-dollar trainer, some-one who would monitor you every day and come up with the perfect exercise designed exactly for your body? A trainer devoted exclu-sively to you, who is continually tweaking your plan to accommodate exactly where you are today? Would you listen to that trainer...or just follow your friends over to spin class?

Well, my dear friend, I am not that trainer—but you are. I'm going to show you how to design a training program that is perfect for you, and I'm going to show you how to keep it perfect for you for the rest of your life—a program that your body loves and that keeps your body strong and lean. Better yet, I'm going to show you how to test your exercise routines to see how they affect your thyroid, your metabolism, and your weight so that you will always be able to find out whether the exercise you're doing is the exact right choice for your unique body. In other words, I'm going to show you how to take this data and create the best possible exercise program for your body.

I'm also going to clear up a lot of exercise myths so that you can find what truly works for you. Maybe you've been avoiding exercise because you just don't have time or think that you can't possibly do enough. No worries! You may find that your ideal exercise is as little as 6 to 8 minutes every other day!

Have you been dreaming of becoming ripped and lean but have been frustrated by weight gain, injuries, and fatigue? Those days are over. You're going to find your own personal path to greater fitness, a path uniquely geared to your body's chemistry. Are you already an athlete but want to get stronger and leaner? The answers all lie ahead.

I am going to help you achieve your dream body and best health ever—in a way that is probably pretty different from what you are doing now. That's because this approach has you testing every single aspect of your exercise plan—which type of exercise you do, when, and for how long—so that you can always be certain that you are doing what is optimal for you. That's what I mean by "million-dollar trainer"—and that's what you are about to become.

Too Little...or Too Much?

Whether you're an over-exerciser or a couch potato, you'll probably be surprised to find out which types of exercise actually are good for you—and how little time you need to get terrific results. The key is to find the sweet spot—the program designed by you. In this chapter, you're going to learn how to do just that.

But first I'd like to share with you two very different success stories. Come meet the woman who exercised too little...and the couple who exercised too much.

Maria: "I don't have time to go to the gym!"

Maria came to me in tears. After more than three years of weight gain, exhaustion, and depression, she had been diagnosed as hypothyroid. Her symptoms had begun when she was promoted to her dream job, which had meant more responsibility and even less time for herself. She loved the work but felt torn about how to get everything done, especially since she had two kids with afterschool activities and a husband who worked late.

Maria knew that she should exercise, but her days were already packed to the gills. "I don't have time to get to the gym and exercise an hour a day, five days a week," she told me. "Some days it seems like I barely have time to shower! By the time weekends come along I'm exhausted and I want to spend time with my family. Plus, I feel selfish going to the gym when there are so many other things that need doing. I feel like such a failure!"

Sound familiar? So many people think it's all or nothing, that if they aren't pumping away in the gym for hours every week, they won't get the benefits of exercise at all. So listen to me, and listen well: I want you to kick that thinking to the curb.

Exercising too intensely will actually make it harder for you to lose weight. As you'll see in this chapter, when you stress your body with exercise that isn't right for your unique chemistry and genetics, your body fights back. Your thyroid struggles, your metabolism slows to a crawl, and basically, nobody is happy.

On the other hand, doing the right exercise for your body is one of the best things you can do. The right types of exercise *for you* will boost your energy, help you lose weight, and make you fit and lean. Your thyroid will perk right up. Your metabolism will start humming at peak speed. You'll feel clearheaded, happy, and ready to take on the world.

To get those fabulous results, you need to find which type of exercise, intensity, and duration work best for your chemistry. It might very well be less intense, quicker, and easier than you think: just 8 to 30 minutes a day, three or four days each week. Most people don't need to exercise more than a total of two hours a week to achieve optimal health and weight. As it happened, that was true for Maria.

"Look, Maria," I told her. "You don't need to kill yourself to be in shape. I want you to go to bed ten minutes earlier so that the next morning, you can do four minutes of warmup and then six minutes of exercises or weight training. You don't even need to buy weights—

you can do body-weighted exercises right in your own bedroom. Your ideal time, to start with, is just two days during the week."

Maria looked at me, almost too surprised to speak.

"On the weekends, if you want, you can go to the gym for your longer workout on Saturdays or Sundays," I continued. "If you're pressed for time, just do an exercise video at home. That will save you even more time. You are *not* a failure. You just needed the right information about exercise when life is stressful."

Maria was still in shock, but she nodded happily and agreed. This small jump start—less than an hour a week—helped to boost Maria's BBT and rev up her metabolism. She was able to lose 16 pounds in one month without ever feeling hungry, exhausted, or overwhelmed. Even better, she was happier, calmer, and more energetic.

Maria liked her new regimen so much, she even got her whole family on board. Her husband and two kids all started exercising at home, and together they worked their way up to 20 minutes, four days a week. I am so proud of her—what a victory!

Dave and Janet: "We exercise all the time. Why are we gaining weight?"

Dave and Janet were one of my favorite couples: motivated, fun-loving folks who adored the thrill of accomplishment and the camaraderie of their CrossFit community. When they first began CrossFit, those challenging workouts seemed like the answer to their prayers. They were having fun, feeling great, and losing weight.

Then, a few months in, each of them began to gain weight. They stopped feeling that wonderful burst of vital energy; instead, they felt fatigued. Each of them started getting injuries, too—a sprained ankle for Dave, an inflamed shoulder for Janet.

At first, they blamed their weight gain on the enforced rest periods from those injuries. But they began to notice other problems. Once vibrant and bubbly, they both began to struggle with anxiety and depression. Instead of getting pumped from exercise, they just felt depleted. They didn't understand what was happening.

"Everyone else we know is doing great on CrossFit!" Dave would say.

"What's wrong with us?" Janet would add.

"Maybe we're not working hard enough?" Dave suggested.

So being the dedicated folks they were, they redoubled their efforts. Oops. More injuries and more weight gain, followed by still more fatigue and lethargy.

Then Janet's hair started to fall out. Her doctor immediately ran a thyroid panel, which showed that Janet's TSH had gone from a normal in-range number of 1.5 to a very out-of-range 4.8. Just in the year she had been doing CrossFit, she had developed full-blown hypothyroidism.

Janet urged Dave to get his blood work done, too. Lo and behold, both his testosterone and his T3 were at disastrous levels. No wonder he was gaining weight and feeling lousy! So both of them came to me, frustrated and confused.

"We know lots of people who do CrossFit," Janet told me.

"Yeah, and everybody else is doing great! Why are we the only ones with health issues?" Dave demanded.

Turns out that CrossFit just wasn't the exercise best suited for them: they were exercising too intensely and for too long. But when I told them to cut back, they fought me on it, as so many exercise lovers do.

"It worked so well at the beginning," Janet insisted.

"How is exercising *less* going to help us lose weight?" Dave wanted to know.

I showed them the data gathered over thousands of patients. Reluctantly, they agreed to try the more varied and less demanding exercise plan that I designed for them—and guess what? Janet lost 10 pounds, and Dave lost 14 in their very first month on The Metabolism Plan. They were doing less exercise and different exercise than they had done before, plus avoiding their reactive foods (whey, turkey, and salmon for Dave; shrimp, spinach, and strawberries for Janet). Six months later, they had each balanced their hormones and were at goal weight, doing an exercise routine they loved.

Where's Your Balance?

The Metabolism Plan helped Dave and Janet find their balance, just as I am going to help you find yours. Remember the story of Goldilocks and the three bears? "Not too little and not too much" needs to be your mantra, too.

When you exercise too little, you're likely to feel sluggish and out of sorts. You find yourself able to do less and less—even carrying your shopping bags to the car seems like an exertion. You sleep restlessly, your inflammation increases, and you tend to gain or retain weight.

When you exercise too much, you may feel fatigued and depleted. You find yourself suffering from mysterious symptoms—hormonal issues, lower sex drive, irritability. You might also face increased inflammation and excess weight because too much physical exertion can read like "Danger!" to your thyroid and immune system.

When you exercise appropriately, though, your stress levels are lower. You feel energized, vigorous, and calm. Your hormones are more balanced, and you lose weight or easily maintain a healthy weight. And for an extra bonus, you have more free time than when you were pushing yourself to overdo it. What you want is just enough physical stress to strengthen your muscles and challenge your body but not so much that you set off your body's danger signals.

How do you find your ideal exercise balance? All you have to do is look at these key factors:

- When you exercise
- How long you exercise
- What kind of exercise you do
- What intensity you choose.

When You Exercise: Timing Is Everything

As with everything else, optimal timing can vary. For most people, though, exercise is better earlier in the day—before work or at lunch.

Why? It's all about the stress. Let's look at two different scenarios so you can see what I mean.

Scenario 1: The Morning Workout

For you, Mondays are a stress bomb, so you aren't about to get up super-early for your workout. Instead, you sleep in a little so you are completely charged and ready to face the day. You do set aside 15 minutes, though, and your morning workout boosts serotonin, leaving you fueled and ready to go.

Monday stresses you out as usual, and when it's over, all you want to do is take it easy. You come home, wind down, and enjoy a great dinner with a glass of wine. After dinner, you talk with friends or maybe spend time with your family, allowing your body to fully relax. You can sleep 15 minutes later tomorrow because you worked out today (you only exercise every other day, to give your body a chance to restore itself). The weekend comes along and if you have more time, you do a longer, more intense workout. Your body is humming along, you are lean and toned, and your thyroid is happy. All is good.

Scenario 2: Working Out After Work

As usual, Monday was a stress bomb—in fact, today seemed a little worse than usual. By the end of the day, your annoying coworkers and your endless commute home have made you feel like a limp dishrag. Exercise to the rescue, right? You want that rush that makes you feel so good—the endorphins (natural painkillers) and serotonin that result from a good workout.

Of course, it's the end of the day, and your body is longing to wind down and relax. (Remember how those cortisol levels drop gradually throughout the day?) But years of listening to the experts has your brain saying, "Spin class!" So you race to the gym to get there on time, replacing your body's natural rhythms with an exercise frenzy. Oops! Sure, you get the endorphin rush from spinning, but guess who is more stressed-out the next day by those coworkers and that commute? You! Especially when you step on the scale and found out you gained a pound! You might *think* that after-work workout feels good, but your body knows better, and it's telling you so every single day, every time you step on the scale.

Daniel, Age 51

I freaked out when Lyn-Genet said that it might be spinning five times a week that was keeping me from losing weight and raising my blood pressure. Spinning is my drug, as I like to say! But sure enough, every time we tested spinning, I gained weight and my BBT dropped. So I did The Metabolism Plan for 30 days, lost 16 pounds, discovered that lamb and steak boosted my thyroid function, and was able to cut my medications. Now that I'm closer to my goal weight I spin just once a week, and that doesn't cause my BBT to drop. I actually have more energy and patience—and hair!—than I used to have.

Beware the Negative Feedback Loop!

There is a phenomenon well-known to stress researchers known as the negative feedback loop. When it comes to stress, it means the more stressed you are, the more stressed you become.

Let's say you're in a jumpy, anxious mood because your cat is sick, you're rushing to the vet, and you have a major work meeting. You're already pretty stressed, and when you get stuck in traffic on the way to work, you feel twice as anxious. If you'd been in a good mood, you might have just shaken your head and shrugged it off. But crazed and keyed up, you find yourself getting really angry. And the next time something upsetting happens—say, a coworker says something mildly annoying—you're *beyond* angry. In other words, the more stressed-out you are, the more you add to your stress.

Now, here's where exercise comes in, because exercise can either disrupt this feedback loop or make it worse. If you exercise *before* you feel super-stressed, you raise your levels of serotonin and decrease your levels of cortisol.

However, if you exercise *while* you're super-stressed, or if you simply exercise too intensely, you push those cortisol levels up too high—so high, they tend to just stay elevated, undermining your sleep and setting you up for a stressful tomorrow where you are also starving all day. Instead of lowering your cortisol levels, exercise actually raises them, creating a bevy of other issues.

"But if I've had a long, rotten day, exercise feels great!" my clients tell me. I get it. Right after you finish your workout, your body is flooded with endorphins and serotonin. These natural feel-good hormones mask your stress and give you one terrific exercise high. Even better, the serotonin acts as a natural antidepressant.

So far, so good—but your cortisol levels are still way up there, at a time of day when they should naturally be dropping. By exercising so late in the day, you are going against the natural flow of your hormones. The endorphins and serotonin are like a drug masking your body's true condition—which is stressed-out, flooded with cortisol, and clinging to excess fat for dear life.

Think of the way a terrific high is often followed by a hangover or a crash. That's you, when you do too much exercise too late in the day. Of course, when you are younger, your body can adapt and repair much more quickly. Now that you're older, your body is less resilient, while you, poor dear, have been beating yourself up for "your body not responding" instead of hearing the message that your body is trying so hard to send.

Now, you might be someone who actually *can* exercise later in the day, so never fear: You'll get to test that, too. You can also try types of exercise that incorporate relaxation and meditation, such as tai chi and yoga.

Sleep Your Way Thin

For most people, working out in the morning or on your lunch hour is best: It fuels you with energy before the stress of the day has depleted you. But please, for the dear love of God, don't compromise sleep so that you can wake up early to exercise, because that totally sets you up to fail. And believe me, few things are worse than killing yourself to get up at 5 a.m. for an early morning workout—and *still* gaining weight.

Have you ever weighed yourself at night and then weighed yourself in the morning? Isn't it amazing that you can lose 2 or 3 pounds sleeping? That's because your body burns the most fat when it's repairing itself—which is what you do when you sleep.

So *please* do not skimp on sleep in order to work out: You'll see a consistently lower BBT, which tells you that your thyroid is struggling. You're setting yourself up for a lousy mood, a loss of energy, disrupted metabolism—and extra weight. Sleep is your secret weight-loss weapon—do not neglect it!

How Long You Exercise: Less Is More

When I first told Janet and Dave that they were exercising too much, they had a hard time believing me. Like everyone else, they loved that exercise high.

But all their intense exercise was also pushing up their cortisol, affecting their hormones, and slowing their metabolism over time. And here's what happens when you've got too much cortisol:

Excess cortisol=
fat storage + skewed hormones + weak adrenals +
malfunctioning thyroid + increased insulin output

Cortisol also causes blood sugar to spike, which can lead to a buildup of blood sugar in your bloodstream. That excess blood sugar in turn triggers a buildup of insulin, which puts you at risk of diabetes and makes it much harder to lose weight.

John first came to me after he was diagnosed with prediabetes at the age of 58. His fasting insulin levels were high—around 20—and his fasting blood sugars were also high, around 110. I like to see fasting insulin less than 6 and fasting blood sugar less than 90, so you can see how out of balance his numbers were. Despite the low-fat diet he had been following for years and the fact that he was exercising five times per week, John could not lose weight, and he could not get his sugar or insulin levels down.

Poor John literally had his metabolism working against him. His intense workouts were dramatically raising cortisol levels—when we tested them, he saw gains every time. This caused his insulin to spike, triggering weight gain.

John was also failing to give his body the low-inflammatory foods he needed. Instead, he loaded up on traditional diet foods like protein powders, egg whites, and spinach. These foods caused him inflammation, which meant that every time he ate he was asking his body to produce more and more insulin to help get this so-called healthy food into his cells. Insulin is also a growth hormone whose job is to pack on fat quickly and efficiently, so the more insulin John was producing, the more weight he was putting on. He was shocked to see his sugar levels rise when he ate these "perfect" foods. As soon as we got John started on The Metabolism Plan, his blood sugars stabilized, his next fasting insulin level dropped to 8 (a dramatic improvement!), he lost 10 pounds within the first three days, and he learned how to exercise in a way that didn't boost his cortisol levels. Problem solved!

Excess insulin and cortisol are not the only problems with overtraining. Too much exercise has been shown to decrease blood levels of several key biochemicals, described in the following list.

- **L-glutamine**: An amino acid that prevents muscle breakdown and improves metabolism. In other words, when over-exercise lowers your L-glutamine levels, you'll find it harder both to build muscles and to lose weight.

- **Dopamine**: A hormone that helps you feel energized and thrilled, as when you ride a roller coaster or fall in love (see page 54). When your dopamine levels are low, you tend to feel listless, unfocused, and unmotivated, as though life has lost its savor.

- **5-HTP**: The precursor to serotonin. While exercise can temporarily increase your serotonin levels—a powerful antidepressant— too much exercise can deplete the very chemical your body needs to make more serotonin. This is why, over time, too much exercise might sabotage your ability to get that exercise high, leaving you depressed and struggling with sleep problems rather than "high" and well rested.

As you can see, we've got a paradoxical effect going on here. In the short term, excess exercise can make you feel great. Over the long haul, however, too much exercise actually sabotages your mood, saps your energy levels, and undermines your body's ability to repair itself. It's similar to the way a quick burst of caffeine or sugar makes you feel energized and happy in the short term—but then, a few hours later, you're crashing. And the more often you repeat those highs, the harder it is to get back to normal, let alone to achieve the 110 percent I want for you.

Exercising too intensely also undermines your hypothalamus and pituitary glands, which your thyroid depends on to function at its peak. So excess exercise compromises your thyroid function and depletes your levels of T3.

In addition, as we saw in Chapter 3, excess cortisol tends to deplete your progesterone and testosterone levels, creating estrogen dominance (true for both men and women!). That creates more thyroid dysfunction and still more weight gain on top of increased moodiness and carb cravings.

Studies show that exercising too intensely for more than half an hour increases hunger, so you often end up eating twice the amount of calories burned. Now, when you consider that your exercise may also slow down your metabolism, you can see how weight gain rather than weight loss is the end result of your workout.

What's Wrong with Cardio?

For years, we've all been told that "cardio" is the golden key to weight loss. Cardio workouts include running, brisk walking, spinning, and aerobics—any vigorous exercise in which your heart rate stays up for extended periods without a break.

But *is* cardio good for weight loss? As you age, the answer is a great big *not really*: Too much cardio can affect your health, your metabolism, and your weight because of the way it creates *oxidative stress.*

Oxidative stress is a normal response to exercise in which your body produces *free radicals*: molecules that are missing an electron. Each free radical seeks to replace its missing electron by pulling it from another molecule. That molecule now has its own unpaired electron, so now it's a free radical, and therefore it, too, seeks to pull an electron from another molecule...and on it goes. Pretty soon, you get a whole bunch of free radicals—and a lot of dysfunctional molecules that can't operate properly because they're each missing an electron.

A free radical's favorite pastime is wreaking havoc in your cells, which is why oxidative stress causes your body to age. Over time, the damage created by oxidative stress increases your risk of heart disease, cancer, type 2 diabetes, and autoimmune diseases.

Free radicals are not inherently bad. Ironically, the more free radicals you have, the more your body is triggered to produce and use *antioxidants*, which combat oxidative stress to make your cells healthy and strong. That's why moderate exercise is actually considered an antioxidant: When you exercise in the right amounts, the stress you cause is the kind that ultimately makes you stronger.

But if you undergo more oxidative stress than your body can handle—more oxidative stress than your antioxidants can combat—then free radicals can overwhelm your cells and you have problems. Big problems, like chronic disease, premature aging, and weight gain.

So when I tell you that long, intense exercise—especially endurance training—can cause excessive oxidative stress, you can see immediately why too much exercise can make you sick, fat, and old before your time. In fact, endurance exercise can increase oxygen usage to 20 times its resting state, which greatly increases your body's level of free radicals. If you don't allow for adequate rest after oxidative stress, you also heighten inflammation, which, as you now know, causes you to gain weight and get sick. We are constantly told "faster, longer, and more intense" when it comes to exercise. But that approach is way less likely to work for us as we age.

Now, that being said, some people are blessed to be athletes. You've seen them—finishing their marathons looking like Greek gods. If *you* are one of those people, you can and probably should do more intense exercise than most. You'll know this because you can eat a healthy, satisfying diet—not a starve-yourself low-cal regime—and continue to maintain a healthy weight, feeling energized and enjoying optimal health while you're maintaining your intense workout routine. Your body knows best, and if your body wants lots of intense exercise, it will tell you!

Most of us, though, need far less exercise than we've been told—especially as we get older. You just need to exercise smarter. It's more likely that the long, intense workouts your body loved when you were younger are now actually hurting you.

Smarter, Not Harder: Appropriate Exercise for You

My goal is to have you active and happy and high functioning right up until your very last breath. I don't buy into this nonsense that says you have to slow down as you get older, and I don't want you to buy into it either. It's just that things change as we age, so we need to find ways to support our body instead of fighting it.

One age-related change is that your body's ability to recover from excess exercise decreases as you get older. As a result, the exercise that worked for you in your 20s might now appear to your body as excessive stress—plus your body is no longer as effective in keeping up with the repair. That's why you have to find the intensity and duration of exercise that fits you *now*, keeping your current body in optimal shape. When you find your own personal bio-individual exercise, your metabolism zips up to peak speed, you can eat normally without gaining weight, and you generally feel terrific.

Don't skip exercise altogether—it really is good for you! Not engaging in regular exercise will slow your thyroid function and deprive you of such health benefits as cardiovascular health and boosts of serotonin, not to mention a terrific natural sleep aid and antidepressant. You just need to find the exercise that works for you.

Julie, Age 37

I've been using Lyn-Genet's approach for almost three years now, and it has become second nature. Starting out at 324 pounds, I never thought I'd ever see the 100s again, and now here I am down to 154 pounds. That's a whopping 170 pounds of weight loss. Crazy, right?!

I finally took control of my life, which was spiraling out of control. I stood up for myself and said, "Never again!" I decided I was important enough to put in the time and effort. I learned my strengths and weaknesses. I've learned not just how to eat, but how to live.

I'm also super excited to start a new journey in my life by working with Lyn-Genet on some exercise videos. It's a little ironic that someone like me will be doing exercise videos. Three years ago, this morbidly obese girl would have laughed in your face if you had said, "You'll be making exercise videos with that woman who wrote the book you're carrying around." Well, I'm not that girl anymore, and I *did* do it. I'm so excited for the possibilities and my new life.

It's amazing to me that I've been able not only to lose the weight but to keep it off. It feels incredible to not be ashamed of my reflection. I used to hide myself from the world. At parties I used to be a wallflower—now I'd say I'm more of a butterfly. In fact, I recently went to a wedding, and aside from eating (which I did without regret), I hardly sat. I danced, I mingled, and I had a blast! Thanks to Lyn-Genet, I'm a new and improved me!

My Story: Running on Empty

Did you know that in my early 30s I was a crazy runner? I ran 50 miles a week, every single week, for years. On top of that? I was working out 6 days a week with heavy weights, and I loved it. Really and truly.

Then my practice started taking off, so I only ran in the spring, and I would work out whenever I got a chance. And my body was still so happy!

But about three years ago, something shifted. My life was a complete stress bomb. And now running started to seem like a chore *and* my body wasn't responding to lifting heavy weights. In fact, I was gaining body fat and weight every time I worked out

I just couldn't believe my "golden" workouts were the problem. Still in shock over what I was seeing with my own eyes, I tested running; that is, I took my BBT and weighed myself the day after I ran.

Well, guess who totally and absolutely failed running? And then weight training with heavy weights? Yup, yours truly. I had a hard time believing it, so I tested it quite a few times. Always the same results: increased weight, decreased BBT. So I took a year off and played tennis. I never would have guessed, and to be honest, I am truly awful at tennis. But I'm having the time of my life, and my body shows me how just much it loves this crazy sport.

P.S. Stress has been really low the last year, so I decided to test running again a few months ago. I discovered that my body still hates the long runs but it now loves sprinting! So these days I go for weekly sprints with my son, bonding, having the time of my life, and feeling great. The heavy weight training? My body loves it again. As long as you listen to your body, you can't go wrong.

What Kind of Exercise: The Right Workout for You

There's only one way to be absolutely sure about which type of exercise is right for you, and that's to test it. In the next 30 days you're going to test your workout and keep testing it, so that you can be 100 percent sure that it's exactly the type, length, and timing of exercise that is perfect for your body. The great news? What you are learning now is the same format you can use for the rest of your life to figure out what works best for you. So if you start The Metabolism Plan in your 20s, you will always know what to eat and how to exercise for now and for the next 70 years.

What tends to work for most people over the age of 35 is to alternate increased and decreased heart rate, an approach known as *interval training*. Rather than running, spinning, or stepping for an hour or more nonstop, you engage in a type of exercise that incorporates both "up" and "down" times, such as weight training, body-weighted movement (where you use your own body's weight rather than a free weight or machine), cardio (in short intervals), and plyometrics, a type of exercise in which you get your muscles to exert maximum force in short bursts. A routine that includes stretching, tai chi, yoga, or Pilates—movement that supports core strength, flexibility, and balance—is also optimal.

More stressful types of exercises cause most people to gain weight or to have trouble losing, especially if they're over 35. I'm talking about spinning, CrossFit, boot camp–style classes, marathons, and Bikram yoga. As Dave and Janet discovered, these types of workouts seem to tip the balance from the perfect amount of stress into too much stress for most bodies.

That being said, you are wonderfully unique! It may be that spinning and CrossFit totally rock your body. Remember: There is no perfect exercise, just what's perfect for *you*. When you begin your 30 days, we'll start you off with the least inflammatory types and times for exercise—the ones that tend to work for everybody. After that, feel free to experiment to find out whether the more intense types are right for you.

Allie, Age 63

For the last few years, I have blamed my bad knees and hips for not exercising, but Lyn-Genet wouldn't hear it. "The good news," she said, "is that you haven't exercised for a long time, so you don't need to do much—but you do need to move!" So she started me off with 6 minutes of low-impact cardio and body-weighted yoga routines. Frankly, I thought she was crazy, but she gets results, so I did it. You know what? I felt better. In a few weeks we added in some more exercises to strengthen and add muscle mass. Now? I feel amazing and stronger. I can carry my groceries, walk upstairs, and get up and down from a chair with no issues. I admit I was daunted thinking I needed to work out super-hard to see real results, and that kept me from exercising at all. Lyn-Genet got me past that idea. I am now seeing results, and I am so excited about it that I've actually started a fitness club with my friends.

Rotate or React

Even when you've found your perfect exercise, you might want to change things up. You've already heard our office's favorite saying: "rotate or react." Whenever you do something too often—whether it's eating the same food every day or repeating the same workout for several months—you risk triggering a negative reaction. For food, that reaction is inflammation, symptoms, and weight gain. For exercise, it's a plateau.

A plateau is when the exercise that used to work for you is no longer challenging your body. Feeling bored? Going through the motions and working out while answering your iPhone? That's smells like a plateau—and it means less progress.

Suppose you've been doing weight training and you just aren't seeing the results you think you should be. Try yoga for a change. If you've been doing yoga for years, you might do better with kettlebells and running.

You might also need to get creative about the way you vary your routines. If you're used to running for 90 minutes at a time, you might taper down to 30 minutes and add in some body-weighted exercises and yoga. This type of variety will also help you prevent injury and create muscular balance. I spent years directing physical therapy clinics, teaching yoga in my health center, and teaching medical massage therapy, so I learned a lot about why people run into problems. The number one cause of injury? Muscular imbalance and overtraining the same muscle groups.

Your body needs change for it to respond. Here are some ways to switch things up and bust through a plateau.

- **Rotate your exercise to a new type**: Switch from Pilates to kettlebells, from running to tennis, from weight training to yoga. Maybe the type of training you're doing now isn't optimal for your body, or you just need a break.
- **Change intensity**: If you're lifting weights, add or decrease weight. If you're moving, move faster. If you're working out in intervals, make the "active interval" a little longer, or shorter and more intense. Find some way to push yourself to switch it up.
- **Change frequency**: If you were doing 12 reps, bump it up to 15. If you're doing 15 at a low weight, try 12 at a heavier weight. Increase or decrease sets and repetitions. If you were working out only two or three days a week, make it four. (However, do not exercise more than four days a week just yet; you can test that later. For now, please continue to alternate one vigorous day with at least one day of restoration.)

Because your body is in a constant state of flux and always responds best to new stimuli, you would ideally rotate your workouts every season. For example, in the spring, you might make your main activity running, then switch to swimming in the summer. In the fall, take up yoga, and in winter try weight training to prepare you for your spring runs. You'll create muscular balance, avoid plateaus, and just plain have more fun. You'll also lower your risk of repetitive stress injuries. So be ready to keep changing, and your body will thank you for it.

Frank, Age 56

I've been running since my teens, and I became a vegetarian in my 20s. I never had a weight issue but always had high cholesterol. But so did my dad and brother, so I just thought it was genetic.

In my 30s, I started having some depression, but I chalked it up to my work, which is pretty stressful and demanding. I started taking antidepressants, but they just weren't helping that much. My cholesterol got so high that my doctor wanted to put me on Lipitor. On my first day working with Lyn-Genet, I checked my BBT. I couldn't believe that it was all the way down to 93! No wonder I was depressed.

As I tested foods, I found that my body needed to switch from a total vegetarian diet. I also discovered that fish and chicken boosted my BBT, so I added it to my diet just a few times a week. I decided to switch up my exercise, too, running only in the spring and summer so my body could get a break for six months. Now I lift weights and do boxing when it gets cold. My weight is healthy, my cholesterol is normal, and my depression is gone. Who knew that such simple steps could change my life?

Does Walking Count as Exercise?

Well, yes...and no. If you live in a suburb and never walk any farther than to the car parked in your driveway, a moderately paced 20-minute walk is *huge*. Yes, that will be exercise, and very beneficial exercise, too, so start a walking club with your family or friends, or make this time a moving meditation for you to decompress.

But if you're even a little bit fit, then no, walking may not count as effective exercise if it's done for less than 20 to 30 minutes. And here's the rub: Walking for more than 20 to 30 minutes might actually be perceived by your body as stress! I have actually seen clients gain a pound just from walking or doing a gentle hike for an hour! So once again, think twice about what you have been told is healthy and listen to the messages your body is giving you.

The other problem with walking is that it might not be challenging enough. Once you're conditioned enough to walk briskly for 20 minutes, you're probably getting only minor benefits. Sure you get some mild cardiovascular support, me time, and vitamin D, but I want you to get maximum payback for your time. For most people in moderately good condition, walking is not an optimal mode of weight loss.

Let's be clear: I don't want you to stop walking! On The Metabolism Plan, you're going to work out every other day, and if you are new to walking, that will be your workout, even if you have to build up to two or three 10-minute walks each day, such as strolling from your car to the other end of the parking lot.

If you are conditioned, you can easily walk 20 minutes a day—but that won't count as exercise, because your body won't perceive it as exercise! I love when my clients take a walk outside at lunchtime. It gets you out of your everyday routine and you get a good healthy dose of vitamin D, all of which is terrific for your thyroid, hormones, and immune function.

Now, you might very well be one of those people who can walk more—what is true for most people may not be true for you. One of my favorite couples are professional dog walkers in Massachusetts. Jerri lost 50 pounds, and her husband, Jack, lost 100 just doing The Metabolism Plan and walking their dogs for the workout. So these are walking "rules" that you will modify to find what makes you happiest and healthiest.

However, if you are stalling in weight loss on the days you walk your dog, here's a simple trick: Bring a Frisbee or a ball and run your dog, letting it fetch while you throw! That way you can keep *your* actual walking to 20 minutes total.

Testing Your Workout: How to Find Your Sweet Spot

As with food testing, you're relying on two simple tools: your scale and your thermometer.

Your Thermometer, a.k.a. Your Thyroid Monitor

Your thermometer will tell you in just two minutes whether your particular workout routine is boosting or depleting your thyroid function. Every morning for your 30 days, you will take your BBT. Check back to page 45 in Chapter 2 for step-by-step instructions on how to do this. Your BBT will tell you how your thyroid is functioning and how sleep, stress, and exercise have affected it and your metabolism. When your BBT goes out of range, you know something didn't work for your body. When it's optimal, you're right on track!

What's Your Range?

- Optimal BBT: 97 to 97.3
- Functional: 96.5 to 97.3
- Above 97.3: Likely to exhibit more hyperthyroid symptoms, such as anxiety, irritability, sleeplessness, and racing heart
- Below 96.5: Likely to exhibit hypothyroid symptoms, such as lethargy, depression, constipation, and weight gain

Women: Please note that your BBT rises when you ovulate and five days or so before your cycle starts. You will need to get 30 days' worth of readings to learn exactly how much.

Your Scale, a.k.a. Your Reality Check

I know many of you out there hate the scale. But once you see how much it can enhance your weight loss and give you valuable information, you're going to love it as much as I do. After all, you deserve to know how the foods you ate and the exercise you engaged in affect your weight—and without the scale, how are you going to find out? If thick-crust pizza doesn't work for you, but thin-crust does, wouldn't you want to know? That's what the scale tells you. You'll also like finding out which exercise your body loves so much that it responds with some extra weight loss.

When your scale goes down (or remains at your healthiest weight), you know that you can safely enjoy the foods and exercise of the previous day. Weight loss means that what you ate or how you exercised did *not* provoke an inflammatory response. Weight gain or weight stabilization (before you've reached your healthy weight) means that you're off track, creating inflammation instead of healing it.

Scale + Thermometer = Success

If you lose a pound the day after you go for a 30-minute run and your BBT is in a functional zone, you have found your sweet spot. If you gain a pound when you do a 30-minute run and your BBT drops, you know you've gone too far. Either way, you've scored a win, because you've just gathered data on what your body wants and needs to achieve and maintain an ideal weight and metabolism.

Example 1: You weigh 170 pounds and your BBT is 96. You test a 30-minute run and the next day you weigh 169.1 pounds and your BBT is 96.8. Bravo, that's a win!

Example 2: You weigh 170 pounds and your BBT is 96. You test a 30-minute run and the next day you weigh 170.8 and your BBT is 95.5. Your run hindered short-term weight loss and slowed your metabolism. That's not why you exercise!

So for the next 30 days, you are going to track your response to exercise every single day and find what your body loves. The more data you accumulate, the more you'll learn about your optimal exercise.

The Metabolism Plan Formula for Testing

The Metabolism Plan lasts for 30 days:

- On the even-numbered days, you'll test your foods. You'll know that a food has passed if you lose at least half a pound that day.
- On the odd-numbered days, you will test your exercise. You'll know that an exercise has passed if you lose at least half a pound that day.

To test exercise, start with your baseline: the least amount of time that counts as exercise, given your current level of conditioning. For some of you, that will be six- to eight-minute brisk walks. For others, it will be a more vigorous workout.

Whatever your starting point is, test it. If you do well—losing at least half a pound and your BBT doesn't drop—then move on to test a different exercise on your next exercise day.

If you don't do well—if you lose less weight than you have been losing, if your BBT drops—then repeat the test on your next exercise day. If you still don't do well, give that same exercise a third try two days later. Remember, you are always exercising one day and then resting a day.

What if your BBT is stable? If you're in the optimal zone, your body loves this exercise. If you aren't in the optimal zone, try increasing and decreasing time to get your BBT in the 97 to 97.3 range.

Why do you test each type and amount of exercise three times? Because if your weight stays the same or goes up, that might not be a negative response to the exercise—it might be caused by some other factor, such as diet, sleep, or stress. In order to know that an exercise works for you, you need to consistently see your BBT in the optimal range while you lose at least 0.5 pound.

When you move on to the next phase, you can bump up your exercise time or intensity for any exercise that works for you. If it works at the new level, great! Find something new to test. If it doesn't, be prepared to test it up to two more times, again, to be sure that your body is responding to the exercise and not to some other factor.

Here's how it might go.

- **The Cleanse (Days 1 to 3)**: No exercise.
- **Laying the Groundwork (Days 4 to 10)**: On Days 5, 7, and 9 you might test, say, weight training for 15 minutes.
- **Stepping It Up (Days 11 to 20)**: On Days 11, 13, 15, and 17, you bump up your exercise time by 20 percent, to 18 minutes. On day 19, increase by another 20 percent, to 22 minutes. This is the sweet spot for most people over the age of 35.
- **Fine-Tuning Your Plan (Days 21 to 30)**: On Days 21 and 23, you can stay at your current level or increase exercise by 20 percent. On Days 25, 27, and 29, test what happens if you exercise two days in a row or for up to 90 minutes. Or, if you'd rather test some other type of exercise scenario, you'll have the chance to do that, too. You also have the option of staying at the same level and increasing, or changing your type of exercise, sometime in the next few months.

Frieda, Age 44

I had been overweight yet eating healthy for years, and nothing seemed to work. Tired of beating myself up in the gym, one day, I just gave up and stopped exercising.

Then my knees started to ache. I went to my doctor for a yearly checkup and heard more bad news. My bone density was bad, and my cholesterol was through the roof.

I knew I had to do something. My dad had died of a heart attack, and I didn't want to go the same way. I was really grasping for answers. My brother had worked with Lyn-Genet and told me that if you didn't want to be a gym rat, you didn't need to be. I thought it was worth a shot. Boy, was it ever! My cholesterol dropped 40 points in 30 days, I lost 14 pounds, and the exercise was so easy!

The Metabolism Plan works. I can do the exercise that works for me, and it's easy. Sure, it took some effort in the beginning, but I wanted this to be the last diet I would ever be on. And it is! I have finally found something that works for me.

Testing Exercise: What It Looks Like

My client Jenny desperately wanted to lose the weight that had started piling on in her 30s. Like clockwork, she had put on 4 or 5 pounds every year, so by the time she came to me she was 48 pounds over her goal weight, with high blood pressure and higher stress levels.

I asked Jenny what she ate. "Oh, healthy foods only!" she assured me. There she was, eating oatmeal every morning and skipping a real lunch in favor of a green juice or a raw kale salad. Her dinners were just as "healthy": turkey burgers, salmon, and quinoa.

These are all highly reactive foods, plus she was slowing her metabolism every time she skipped her lunch. Your body experiences a missed meal as starvation—time to slow down your metabolism! Topping it all off was Jenny's 5:30 a.m. boot camp, which meant that she often lost sleep, given all the attendant stress on her thyroid and imbalance in her hunger and fullness hormones.

Then Jenny started the cleanse, which doesn't allow you to work out for the first three days. Suddenly, for someone who couldn't lose a pound, Jenny saw that the weight was flying off. She lost 5 pounds, and her BBT rose from 94 to 96! Better yet, she had more energy and was feeling less stressed.

On Day 5, you start to exercise, but I want you to start slowly so you can establish a baseline—the way your body reacts at the level of exercise that fits your current conditioning. Jenny was an intermediate exerciser, so her starting point was 12 minutes—much less than she was used to. Along with this less intense workout, Jenny was getting way more sleep than before. Lo and behold, her BBT was rising every day and her weight continued to drop. Jenny was finally supporting her thyroid and her body with the food and exercise that were right for her.

Exercising only every other day, Jenny said she had never felt better in her life. She was more patient at work and with her kids, and she felt great about her consistent weight loss of 0.5 pound a day and 0.8 pound on successful workout days. She loved her newfound vitality, which made her feel as though she had left behind her stressed-out, overscheduled life and was now allowing herself to have more "me" time and family time. After just 20 days of nonreactive foods, moderate exercise, and sufficient sleep, Jenny had lost 11.2 pounds and her BBT was in a functional zone of 97!

Day 21 is when you start to test more intense exercise, so Jenny decided to test her beloved 5:30 a.m. boot camp. The results couldn't have been clearer. Jenny's BBT dropped to 95.5, and she gained a pound her first day. Like most of us, Jenny had a hard time believing that something so supposedly healthy could actually slow your metabolism and cause you to gain weight. So she tested that class again, two more times. Both times, epic fail.

"How do you think the boot camp would affect me if I didn't lose sleep?" Jenny asked me. So we tested it on the weekends, when she got to sleep in. The extra sleep kept her BBT from dropping as much, but she still couldn't lose an ounce doing boot camp.

It turned out that Jenny's body did better with barre, a set of ballet-like exercises that build strength and flexibility while using a bar attached to the wall. In that class, she discovered a community of people she liked, and she loved the exercise. The solution for Jenny was simple. On Tuesdays and Thursdays, she did 12 to 20 minutes of weights and plyometrics, and then a nice long barre class on Saturdays. I just got a happy email from her: She's lost 55 pounds in five months.

Here's the lesson Jenny learned—and the most important thing for you to remember: Your body is perfect—and it talks to you every day. You should never be tired, you should never be stressed to the max, and there is no reason on earth you should be putting on weight from exercise. The Metabolism Plan gives you all the tools you need to understand what your body is saying daily. You will learn to turn off that brain in your cranium and start trusting the brain in your gut. A whole new world of weight loss, energy, and health will be your reward.

Part Two

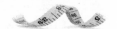

HEAL YOUR METABOLISM IN 30 DAYS

CHAPTER SIX

What You Need to Know Before You Start

The Metabolism Plan is really easy if you have everything ready to go. On the other hand, scrambling for items at the last minute can get those stress levels up. So in this chapter, you're going to learn exactly how to lay the groundwork for success. Your 30 days will go smoothly if you can take a few days before beginning to put your starter kit together, get your kitchen all set up, and make sure you understand exactly how your Metabolism Plan is going to work.

Let's get the logistics out of the way, so you can focus on your success.

Your Metabolism Plan Starter Kit

You need just a few items to start your Metabolism Plan. Each is relatively inexpensive and easy to find. Have these ready to go before Day 1 of your Plan.

• **A digital bathroom scale**: Every morning, you're going to weigh yourself so that you can find out whether the previous day's food and exercise are things your body likes. I know that over the years, you've learned to hate the scale, but starting today, the scale is your new best friend. Not only will you be losing weight quickly; you'll love the information that the scale provides. If your weight goes down, you've done something that works for your body. If it goes up, you've done something that doesn't work, at least right now. If you stabilize, you are moderately reactive and you won't have that food during your 20 days. I would suggest waiting to retest that food after your 20 days when you start to make your own menus. A reliable scale that measures your weight precisely will give you the best possible information about what is going on with your body, as well as alerting you to any sources of inflammation that might be driving your weight upward.

You want a digital scale that is more accurate than one that just measures to 0.1 pound because even a 0.2-pound deviation can have huge ramifications for your data. I recommend the EatSmart Precision Premium digital scale, which runs about $35.

Do you think your current scale is good enough? Then do me a favor. Step on and off it four times. If you get the exact same reading every time, you are fine! But if it gives you a different number even once, you are going to need a better scale. I don't want you to put in all this commitment and get inaccurate information!

• **A digital thermometer**: If your scale helps you measure your degree of inflammation, your thermometer helps you gauge your thyroid function. As we saw in Chapter 2, you'll be taking your temperature every morning to see how your thyroid is responding to your diet, exercise, sleep, and stress. No waiting for your blood work to come back from the lab—the thermometer means you can find out instantly how your thyroid is doing.

• **Cooking utensils**: No need to get fancy here, either. During your first 30 days on The Metabolism Plan, you'll whip up delicious food that's surprisingly quick and easy, so that your focus can be on testing food and exercise. Later, if you like, you can cook elaborate gourmet meals (and you can find some great recipes in *The Plan Cookbook*, too!). However, don't underestimate how delicious "quick and easy" can be. I can't tell you how many people have taken the recipes from the first 30 days and used them for dinner parties!

The list of what you need is short and sweet:

- large sauté pan or wok
- roasting pan or large baking dish
- soup pot
- grater
- sharp un-serrated knife.

I also recommend the following three optional items.

- **Crock-Pot**: Great when you're pressed for time. You can make your soups in it, and you can even roast a whole chicken. (See page 272.)
- **Spiralizer**: A handy little device that creates long spiral swirls out of vegetables like zucchini. Spiralizer-zucchini pasta is super fun and easy to make, and a spiralizer will run you only $15 to $30. Zucchini pasta tastes even better after four or five days, so feel free to use your spiralizer to make a big batch and then keep it in the fridge for the week. If you don't want to invest in a spiralizer, just sub in sautéed yellow squash or zucchini on the days that call for zucchini pasta.
- **A notebook, journal, or weight-loss tracking sheet from my website, www.lyngenet.com**: It's vital to keep a record of the data you collect, since that will be the blueprint for your new way of life. You can do it by hand, or keep your weight-loss tracking sheet handy on your computer to update daily. Here's what the tracking sheet looks like.

YOUR METABOLISM PLAN WEIGHT-LOSS TRACKING SHEET	
Health goals for the next 30 days	
Weight goals for the next 30 days	
Supplements you are on	
Reactive foods	
Friendly foods	
Foods to retest	

NOTE: Always list your weight with the number of the day before. Your weight is a reflection of what you ate the day before.

Date	Which day was yesterday?	This morning's weight	This morning's BBT	Hours you slept last night	Water intake yesterday (include tea)	Exercise you did yesterday (type, duration)	Comments—please list 1. What was tested 2. Any physical symptoms of a reactive response 3. Stress levels
	Day 0 Your first day on The Metabolism Plan						
	Day 1						
	Day 2						
	Day 3						
	Day 4						
	Day 5						
	Day 6						
	Day 7						
	Day 8						
	Day 9						
	Day 10						
	Day 11						
	Day 12						
	Day 13						
	Day 14						
	Day 15						

Day 16						
Day 17						
Day 18						
Day 19						
Day 20						
Start self-designed meal plans—note details **Day 21**						
Day 22						
Day 23						
Day 24						
Day 25						
Day 26						
Day 27						
Day 28						
Day 29						
Day 30						

Your 20-Day Eating Plan

Starting on Day 21 you will be making your own menus, but I wanted to give you a quick idea of what the next 20 days will look like:

DAY 1

BREAKFAST

Flax Granola (page 251) with ½ cup blueberries
Served with Silk Coconut Milk or Rice Dream

LUNCH

Carrot Ginger Soup (page 252)
Sautéed or steamed broccoli
Baby romaine with fresh herbs of choice and sunflower seeds,
    dressed with EVOO, lemon juice, and herbs of choice

SNACK

1 medium-sized apple

DINNER

Kale with Spicy Coco Sauce (page 271) with sunflower seeds
Beet and Carrot Salad (page 257) with pumpkin seeds, lemon
    juice, EVOO, and your choice of herbs

DAY 2

BREAKFAST

Flax Granola (page 251) with pear
Served with Silk Coconut Milk or Rice Dream

LUNCH

Carrot Ginger Soup (page 252) with sunflower seeds

Baby romaine with ¼ avocado, EVOO, lemon juice, and herbs of
   choice
Sautéed or steamed broccoli

SNACK

Apple and almonds

DINNER

Kale with Spicy Coco Sauce
Basmati rice with pumpkin seeds
Beet and Carrot Salad (page 257) with sunflower seeds, lemon
   juice, and EVOO

DAY 3

BREAKFAST

Flax Granola (page 251) with apple
Served with Silk Coconut Milk or Rice Dream

LUNCH

Baby romaine with grated carrots, ¼ apple, and sunflower seeds,
   dressed with EVOO, lemon juice, and herbs
Cream of Broccoli Soup (page 253)

SNACK

Spicy Roasted Pumpkin Seeds (page 267)

DINNER

Chicken with herbs or spices of choice
Roasted Vegetables (page 256)
Baby romaine with avocado, EVOO, lemon juice, and herbs

DAY 4

BREAKFAST

Flax Granola (page 251) with friendly fruit of choice (page 14)
Served with Silk Coconut Milk or Rice Dream

LUNCH

Roasted vegetables, reheated and served on a bed of baby romaine
with pumpkin seeds, along with hard or soft goat cheese

SNACK

Carrots with raw almond butter
OR
Trail Mix

DINNER

Chicken with herbs or spices of choice
Baby romaine with carrots and avocado
Zucchini Pasta (page 256) with Sunflower Pesto (page 262)

DAY 5

BREAKFAST

TMP Smoothie (page 248)

LUNCH

Baby romaine with radicchio, grated raw beet, and pumpkin
seeds
Cream of Broccoli Soup (page 253)

SNACK

Carrots with raw almond butter
OR
Bare brand Apple Chips OR Apple Chips (page 269)

DINNER

Chicken with Spicy Apricot Glaze (page 263)
Sautéed zucchini with onion, basil, lemon juice, and Manchego
Baby romaine with pomegranate

DAY 6

BREAKFAST

Flax Granola (page 251) with friendly fruit of choice
  (page 14)
Served with Silk Coconut Milk or Rice Dream
OR
Blueberry Compote (page 249)

LUNCH

Baby romaine with leftover zucchini, avocado, pumpkin seeds,
  and Manchego
Lemon Basil Escarole Soup (page 254)

SNACK

1 ounce Bare Apple Chips OR Apple Chips (page 269)
OR
Trail Mix (page 267)

DINNER

Your choice of grilled steak, lamb, wild whitefish (preferably
  halibut or flounder), or duck breast; OR eggs with kale and
  broccoli (portion sizes are on page 166)
Roasted Vegetables (page 256)
Baby romaine with ¼ avocado and herbs of choice

DAY 7

BREAKFAST

Flax Granola (page 251) with friendly fruit of choice (page 14)
Served with Silk Coconut Milk or Rice Dream
OR
Apple Streusel (page 249)

LUNCH

Leftover roasted vegetables, reheated and served on a bed of
baby romaine with almond slivers
Cream of Broccoli Soup (page 253)

SNACK

1 ounce salt-free potato chips with Zucchini Noush (page 269)
OR
Trail Mix (page 267)

DINNER

Chicken with fresh herbs or approved spices (page 139)
Sautéed vegetables: Broccoli, yellow squash, and scallions
Baby romaine and grated carrots

DAY 8

BREAKFAST

TMP Smoothie (page 248)

LUNCH

Sautéed vegetables on a bed of baby romaine with almond slivers
Chicken Kale Soup (page 254)

SNACK

Trail Mix (page 267)
OR
Spicy Roasted Pumpkin Seeds (page 267)

DINNER

Test a new protein—beef, lamb, wild whitefish, duck breast, or eggs
Zucchini Pasta (page 256) sautéed with scallions and topped with
grated Manchego
Baby romaine with grated carrot and herbs of choice

DAY 9

BREAKFAST

Flax Granola (page 251) with friendly fruit of choice (page 14)
Served with Silk Coconut Milk or Rice Dream

LUNCH

Sautéed kale with TMP Caesar dressing (page 266), avocado,
apple, and pumpkin seeds
Lemon Basil Escarole Soup (page 254) or Carrot Ginger Soup
(page 252)

SNACK

Low-sodium potato chips (1 ounce)
OR
Trail Mix (page 267)

DINNER

Any friendly protein (to help you choose, see "Rotate or React:
The Protein Story" on page 175; portion sizes on page 166)
Leftover roasted vegetables
Baby romaine with grated carrots and herbs of choice

DAY 10

BREAKFAST

Flax Granola (page 251) with approved fruit of choice
(see page 14)
Served with Silk Coconut Milk or Rice Dream

LUNCH

Cream of Broccoli Soup (page 253)
Baby romaine with almond slivers and carrots

SNACK

Spicy Roasted Pumpkin Seeds (page 267)
OR
Trail Mix (page 267)

DINNER

Your choice of a new protein: grilled steak, lamb, wild whitefish
(preferably halibut or flounder), duck breast, venison, scallops,
lentils, tempeh, or pinto beans on a bed of romaine; OR eggs
Sautéed kale, yellow squash with scallions, and grated Manchego

DAY 11

BREAKFAST

Flax Granola with approved fruit (see page 251)
Served with Silk Coconut Milk or Rice Dream
OR
Almond Grabbers (page 266) and approved fruit

LUNCH

Baby romaine with hard or soft goat cheese, carrots, and dried
cranberries
Cream of Broccoli Soup (page 253)

SNACK

Trail Mix (page 267)
OR
Low-sodium potato chips

DINNER

Chicken with herbs of choice
Sautéed Zucchini Pasta (page 256) and Sunflower Pesto (page 262)
Baby romaine with radicchio and pomegranate

DAY 12

BREAKFAST

TMP Smoothie (page 248)
OR
Blueberry Compote (page 249)

LUNCH

Chicken Kale Soup (page 254)
Baby romaine with avocado and pumpkin seeds

SNACK

1 ounce Bare Apple Chips OR Apple Chips (page 269) with
    optional Zucchini Noush (page 269)
OR
Trail Mix (page 267)

DINNER

Any protein you have tested and found friendly
Test a new vegetable—sautéed, steamed, or baked
Sautéed zucchini, yellow squash, and scallions
Baby romaine and pomegranate

DAY 13

BREAKFAST

Flax Granola (page 251) with a friendly fruit (page 14)
Served with Silk Coconut Milk or Rice Dream

LUNCH

Leftover vegetables with sunflower seeds and apple on a bed of
    red leaf lettuce
Chicken Kale Soup (page 254)

SNACK

Trail Mix (page 267)
OR
Low-sodium potato chips

DINNER

Any protein that you have tested and found friendly
Baby romaine with grated carrots and herbs of choice
Sautéed kale and carrots

DAY 14

BREAKFAST

Any breakfast you have tested and found friendly
OR
Test bread with raw almond butter and apple
OR
Test Arrowhead Mills Spelt Cereal, with chia seeds and sunflower
    seeds (for portion, see page 166)

LUNCH

Chicken Kale Soup (page 254)
Baby romaine with sunflower seeds and carrot

SNACK

1 ounce low-sodium potato chips
OR
Trail Mix (page 267)

DINNER

Approved protein (see page 166)
Zucchini Pasta (page 256) with scallions, basil, and grated Man-
    chego (for portion, see page 166)
Baby romaine with pear

DAY 15

BREAKFAST

Blueberry Compote (page 249)
OR
TMP Smoothie (page 248)

LUNCH

Cream of Broccoli Soup (page 253)
Baby romaine with grated raw beet and pumpkin seeds

SNACK

Carrots with Vegan Creamy Kale Dip (page 270)
OR
Trail Mix

DINNER

Chicken (page 272) with Indian Spice Rub (page 258)
Sautéed kale with onions and yellow squash
Baby romaine and pomegranate

DAY 16

BREAKFAST

Flax Granola with friendly fruit (see page 251)
Served with Silk Coconut Milk or Rice Dream

LUNCH

Chickpea option: Sautéed chickpeas with curry, carrots, and kale
Baby romaine with avocado and sunflower seeds
OR
Rice option: Sautéed kale with yellow squash with basmati rice,
    topped with pumpkin seed hummus (page 268)
Salad with grated beet and carrot

SNACK

Low-sodium potato chips
OR
Almond Grabbers (page 266)

DINNER

Any protein you have tested and found friendly
Steamed, roasted, or sautéed vegetables you have tested and
    found friendly
Baby romaine with radicchio

DAY 17

BREAKFAST

Apple Streusel (page 249)
OR
Blueberry Compote (page 249)

LUNCH

Chicken Kale Soup (page 254)
Baby romaine with avocado, dried cranberries, and sunflower
    seeds

SNACK

Spicy Roasted Pumpkin Seeds (page 267)
OR
Bare Apple Chips OR Apple Chips (page 269) and Zucchini
    Noush (page 269)

DINNER

Friendly protein
Vegetable Timbale (page 257)
Baby romaine with grated beet and herbs of choice

DAY 18

BREAKFAST

TMP Smoothie (page 248)
OR
Blueberry Compote (page 249)

LUNCH

Roasted or steamed broccoli on a bed of baby romaine with carrots, goat cheese, and sunflower seeds
Lemon Basil Escarole Soup (page 254)

SNACK

1 ounce low-sodium potato chips with ⅛ cup homemade guacamole (page 271)

DINNER

Test a restaurant
OR
Choose any friendly dinner you have enjoyed.

DAY 19 AND DAY 20

Repeat your two favorite days so far.

Cooking on The Metabolism Plan

Throughout The Plan, I recommend preparing big batches as often as possible so you'll have lots of leftovers. I also recommend doing as much as you can ahead of time. (As a working mom, believe me, I know the value of time!) For instance, while you are gathering your supplies, try making all your soups and freezing them. After the first few days, you'll be eating chicken every other day, so why not roast a chicken on Day 3 for the whole week? Voilà! Half your kitchen time is done already!

I promise that all of the recipes on The Metabolism Plan are real no-brainers. Remember, the Plan started in New York City, where people have kitchens the size of broom closets! If you ever want to get more elaborate, you can branch out to recipes in *The Plan Cookbook*. But again, for your first 30 days, let's keep it quick and simple.

I want you to be totally confident you have everything you need, so let me answer some frequently asked questions to clear up anything you might be wondering about.

What About Protein?

Adequate protein is crucial to your weight loss and overall health. For the first 20 days, you don't need to do any calculating, because all the meals are carefully calibrated for you. But in case you're curious, I have the day structured so that women have 10 to 40 grams of protein for breakfast, 15 to 25 grams of protein for lunch, and 25 to 60 grams of protein for dinner. Men have 15 to 50 grams for breakfast, 20 to 35 grams for lunch, and 40 to 70 grams for dinner. This is actually a very high-protein diet, but unlike traditional high-protein diets, it's relatively low in meats and high in vegetarian proteins.

Proteins make up the majority of molecules in your body—not just muscle, but also hormones, including insulin, and vital biochemicals, such as enzymes. When you're short on protein for even a single day, you slow your metabolism as your body converts other molecules like glucose and fat into amino acids, which are used to make more protein.

Continued lack of protein also means your body doesn't produce enough enzymes, which causes decreased hormone levels. Enzymes catalyze the vast majority of metabolic reactions in your body—without them, life does not exist! Please support all these components of your body by making sure you get enough protein for the best weight loss and repair.

Do I Need to Buy Organic Produce?

People ask me about this all the time. In an ideal world I would say eat everything organic. But sometimes organic food is not easy to procure or becomes too much of a budget drain. If buying 100 percent organic isn't a viable option, here are a few suggestions.

- Check out the Environmental Working Group website (ewg .org), where you can find two wonderful lists: the "Dirty Dozen" and the "Clean Fifteen." The first is a list of the most pesticide-laden foods—the ones you really should buy organic if you possibly can. The second is of the foods that are relatively clean, even when conventionally grown, so you don't need to be as concerned with buying them organic. These lists change annually, so I suggest you check them once a year.
- Look online. The online market has exploded with organic foods that are inexpensive and can be shipped right to your door.
- Check out Costco and other huge discount stores, which often have an incredible array of organic, hormone-free, antibiotic-free, and wild foods at a fraction of the cost in specialty stores.
- Buy food in season when you can. When you can't, rely on frozen items such as organic blueberries to keep your budget in check.

What About Fish and Meat? Do They Need to Be Organic?

I definitely see people having reactions and gastrointestinal upset to farm-raised fish, which accounts for about 50 percent of the fish currently consumed in the United States. To be frank, the research on the health risks of farm-raised fish is pretty alarming. When you consider the way some of these fish are raised, that's not surprising:

- Some are given large amounts of antibiotics to avoid disease spreading in overcrowded pens.

- Some of their feed contains high levels of PCBs, a hazardous industrial compound.
- Some have been shown to contain high levels of dioxins and mercury, also major toxins that burden your body, stress your thyroid, and overwork your immune system.

Incredible, right? Most people think fish are healthy, but now you know that farmed-raised fish are anything but!

What's the solution? You can sometimes find affordable flash-frozen wild fish. I also buy wild fish when it's on sale and freeze it myself.

For meat, the news is much better: Antibiotic- and hormone-free meat usually costs only a little more than conventional meat, and in the next 30 days you will be consuming a lot less meat than you're probably used to. So even if the meat is a bit more expensive, you'll spend about the same as you did before while also being kinder to the earth's ecosystem. Sounds like a winning scenario to me!

Now, it's not often, but I have seen it: If someone reacts to a particular food, they might also react to animals who eat that food. A prime example is when someone is reactive to corn—they might also be reactive to corn-fed beef, but not to grass-fed beef. It's amazing how sensitive the body can be! This explains why so many people can do great eating grass-fed beef while having an inflammatory reaction to corn-fed. It's not the beef—it's what the beef ate.

Your takeaway: Choose organic and local, absolutely, if you can manage it. If that isn't in your budget, there are a lot of great alternatives for you. Certainly, going antibiotic- and hormone-free is a step in the right direction.

Do I Need to Take Supplements?

Generally, it's best to take supplements only when you need them. However, during the initial stages of The Metabolism Plan, you will be using a few supplements to help your body achieve its optimal noninflammatory state. If you need them, you might also be taking supplements in small doses through the whole 30 days. The goal is to take whatever you need when you need it, let the supplement do its job, then allow your body to heal on its own.

When you start your 30 days, you do want that little nudge, so here's what I recommend.

• **Liver detoxifier**: The liver is responsible for over 500 functions, including regulating metabolism and synthesizing and secreting hormones. I'd love you to support your liver with a morning glass of water and lemon, plus one of the detoxifier choices that I post on my website (www.lyngenet.com). Don't like taking pills? That's okay, you can start with something milder, such as dandelion tea. Whatever you choose, please take it first thing in the morning and remember that if you have it as a tea, it counts toward your total water intake. The liver does a nice job of detoxing while you sleep, so giving it a little extra love in the morning is great for your hormones and your overall health. Once you finish your 30 days, you can let go of the supplement, but please do continue with your morning glass of water and lemon.

• **MSM**: Methylsulfonylmethane, a.k.a. MSM, is a natural form of sulfur that can reset your body's entire histamine response while reducing your reactivity to foods. MSM is a building block of collagen, which you also need for healthy skin, nails, and hair.

If I were a songwriter, I'd write a love song for this fabulous supplement, which has made such a huge difference in my life and the lives of thousands of Metabolism Planners. I first found out about it when I was suffering from awful seasonal allergies that regularly triggered sinusitis and three-day migraines. Finally, I couldn't deal with the pain anymore and did some research. When I discovered MSM, I was thrilled: I took it for six weeks and didn't need to take it again for years. Five years later, I felt that awful pressure in my head and took one dose of 3,000 mg. The pain was gone again for a year! Now, every few years, I might need to take it for a day or two, and my body immediately resets.

It's amazing how often I see people who are severely overweight also suffering from allergies. What's the correlation? Weakened mucosa! We are one long mucosal chain from our sinuses down to our colon. If you have one weak link in the chain, such as asthma, you are likely to have other issues, such as more food sensitivities and weight gain. The major anti-allergy component of MSM works by creating a natural blocking interface between hosts and allergens. Here's something else to consider: Excess histamine can cause anxiety and depression. Plus heightened levels of histamine in the brain stimulate the fight-or-flight response, which can also trigger anxiety. So you can take MSM in response to any of these conditions, and your body will thank you for it.

Why Would You Take MSM on The Metabolism Plan?

- Acid reflux
- Allergies
- Anxiety
- Arthritis
- Asthma
- Candida (intestinal yeast)
- Collagen synthesis for skin, hair, and nails
- Depression
- Inflammation (especially of mucous membranes)
- Leaky gut
- Migraines
- Stress
- Wrinkle reduction

Lucy, Age 31

MSM has been a lifesaver for me. I was using nasal spray nightly in conjunction with allergy meds just so I could sleep. I also had been experiencing anxiety and panic attacks for over a year. I tried St.-John's-wort and it gave me dry mouth while doing nothing to ease the anxiety. I started taking MSM twice a day with no allergy spray or allergy meds. After a week, I was almost anxiety-free and my allergy symptoms were gone soon after. It's amazing!

• **Probiotics**: A supplement that supplies friendly bacteria to replenish your gut. These bacteria are part of your *microbiome*, and they are crucial for your digestion, metabolism, mood, cognitive function, and overall health. Choose a probiotic with many different strains, but make sure it doesn't contain FOS (fructooligosaccharides), which can cause gas and bloating and potentially feed yeast. Your microbiome is vulnerable to reactive foods, stress, insufficient sleep, infections, and any type of gut issue, so a good supply of probiotics will help you maintain optimal digestion and health.

Also, whenever you have a reactive response, a probiotic quickly helps to restore gastrointestinal balance. That means less inflammation and therefore less weight gain. Probiotics also help to ease the constipation that often occurs when you eat a reactive food. Finally, reactive foods promote the growth of yeast, so if you show signs of excess yeast, popping a probiotic is the way to go. The friendly bacteria will help to drive out the yeast, restoring a healthy balance in your gut.

How Do You Know if You Have Excess Yeast?

• You feel gassy and bloated.
• You have a white-coated tongue.
• You crave sweets and starches, sometimes to the point where you feel out of control.

- You experience increased moodiness and inability to concentrate.
- You struggle with heightened hormonal responses such as PMS or menopausal symptoms.

What if I Have Problems with Yeast?

Folks, this is not just a woman's thing! Men have yeast, women have yeast, we all have yeast, which is a fungus that populates our gut.

But when yeast colonies start to overpopulate, you lose the balance of friendly bacteria and yeast, and then you can have issues with your weight, mood, and digestion. Too much yeast can "eat away" at your intestinal wall, allowing partially digested food inside your gut to leak into your bloodstream. Toxins can leak out of your gut, as well. As we have seen, this condition is known as *leaky gut*. Yeast's contribution to leaky gut is a prime reason why obesity, depression, adrenal fatigue, and autoimmune diseases are on the rise.

This is pretty serious stuff, but what if you just have a mild case of yeast overgrowth, as is true for most people? Well, getting even mild yeast overgrowth in check is vital for balanced hormones and optimal digestion. When yeast is rampant, your weight loss stalls. You're crabby, poochy, and craving carbs.

Let's figure out if yeast is an issue for you. Since this fungus feeds primarily on sugar and fermented foods, I want you to do a yeast test the week before you start The Metabolism Plan. Have a nice dinner with some beer, wine, or sparkling cider. Enjoy a lovely salad with one of our vinaigrettes (see page 265), and then top it all off with your favorite dessert. The next morning, before you eat or drink anything, check your tongue in the mirror. If it's coated white, you now know that yeast is an issue for you.

If you do have yeast, don't fret: This is easy to handle, and it's great that we're addressing this now, right? Get some of the probiotics I recommend on The Metabolism Plan website and take them for a few days before you start The Metabolism Plan. You should also start taking MSM, which will prime your body for optimal weight loss and healing. Then, when it's time to enjoy wine and chocolate on Day 4, you will be ready to join the party!

How Much Water Should I Drink?

It is nothing short of incredible how much drinking water affects your ability to lose weight—and to heal. You need water for every metabolic and cellular process that keeps your body alive. When you don't drink enough water, you divert your body's energy from healing. It's as though you are telling your body, "Hey, I'm facing a real drought here, so please stop all of the repair work you would like to do. What I need you to do instead is divert energy allocated for repair and instead extract as much water as you can from all the food I eat. *Then* I want you to hold on to this water in reserve inside my tissues, so I can stay alive."

In other words, when you aren't drinking enough water, you are *retaining* water. Sure, it's just water weight, but what a lousy way to gain weight! Those pounds add up, too, while you feel miserable because your rings aren't fitting and your pants won't button.

You would be astonished if you realized how much weight gain is due to not drinking enough water. Every day I see someone short themselves by even 16 ounces of water and then retain half a pound of water or even more. The wonderful flipside is all the people I see losing 5 to 7 pounds in their first week, just by drinking the amount of water that is right for them!

So how do you determine how much water is right for you? It's very simple. Divide your body weight in half and drink that many ounces each day. That's your base. If you exercise, drink to quench thirst while working out, and in addition, drink your normal amount of water. You're probably going to add about 8 ounces for every 30 minutes of exercise. If you have wine at night, add roughly 4 ounces of water during the day for each glass of wine.

Now, here's your golden rule:

Never drink water after dinner.

Why? That's because it hampers digestion, which means you might wind up stabilizing or even gaining weight. Gaining weight from drinking water is pretty depressing, so please avoid that if you can! I personally do a mental check-in at noon and at 5 p.m. to make sure I'm getting enough water. Then I make sure to finish my last pint at least 45 minutes before dinner. The good news about getting your water in so early? You won't have to get up in the middle of the night to urinate! More sound sleeping means improved metabolism and better weight loss.

What about when it's hot? Hot weather can be tricky, especially because some people retain water when they are out in the heat for too long. The basic rule would be an extra 16 ounces for every 90 minutes you are out being active.

Now, this isn't one of those situations where if something is good, then more of it is better. *Please* don't go over the recommended water amounts, because that can tax your kidney function, making your kidneys less able to process water. And that can mean…yes, you guessed it: water weight gain. So don't think you'll be teacher's pet by drinking more. Stick with what your body needs.

A Few Exceptions

- If you weigh more than 240 pounds or have had gastric bypass, you can decrease your water intake by roughly 20 percent. Most people do well with 110 ounces.
- If you have kidney issues or any other medical issues that require limiting your water intake, please consult your doctor to find out how much you should drink.

Can I Substitute a Food Mentioned on a Menu Plan?

Basically, no, and I'll tell you why. Every single food on The Metabolism Plan is carefully chosen as the least reactive type and amount of food, as well as for its part in creating the most successful food combinations. So please don't deviate. Seemingly small changes can have huge ramifications.

Here's the example that surprises folks the most. I have seen people lose weight with broccoli but gain a pound with broccolini or broccoli rabe. If you thought you were just making a simple substitution and then you gained weight, it would throw off your whole understanding of what your body was doing.

Later on you can test anything you want, including various combinations and portion sizes. But in the beginning, it's just not worth it to throw in extra variables. Let's make sure we're testing just one thing at a time.

If I'm Hungry, Can I Have More Meals?

No, and here's why: I want you eating each meal until you are good and full so that you don't need to graze throughout the day. Instead of adding more meals, don't be shy with your portions!

Three meals and one snack is so much better than five or six mini-meals, for the simple reason that digestion diverts your body's energy from repair. Your body has two choices: It can either digest, or repair itself. Digestion will always take priority. That's why sleep is so important: a long, uninterrupted stretch of time when your body can repair itself without having to bother about digestion.

So, if you are snacking all day, you aren't healing as much—and healing is when you lose the most weight.

Can I Switch Lunch and Dinner if I Need To?

Yes, you can. In fact, if you know you have a long day at work, this can work really well in your favor. Many people have trouble digesting large meals at the end of a stressful day, so try having your dinner meal at lunchtime and your lunch at dinner! Just don't mix and match meals from different days, because the menu plan for each day is chemically balanced. In other words, you can swap Day 6's lunch and dinner, but don't do Day 6's lunch and Day 5's dinner. Stick with one day at a time.

Some people find they experience an energy dip when they have animal protein for lunch. So if you do swap a dinner and lunch on a day when animal protein is called for at dinner, pay attention to your energy levels. If you crash in the midafternoon, that's a sign that animal protein at lunch isn't ideal for you.

Also please avoid soup at night. It's strange, but I always see it hampering weight loss—perhaps because of the water content. So if Cream of Broccoli Soup is called for at lunch and you want to switch your lunch and dinner, just have steamed or sautéed broccoli instead. Voila, problem solved!

Can I Drink Coffee?

Well…. during the cleanse, I'd kind of rather you didn't, and here's why. Coffee is mildly stressful for your body, so it's nice to take a break during the cleanse and concentrate on total healing. Coffee is a great antioxidant, though, so you can bring it back on Day 4 and on with my blessing!

Also, remember how I wanted you to have your body functioning on its own without the use of outside aids? Well, coffee induces peristalsis, the process that enables you to have bowel movements. When your body becomes dependent on outside aids, it stops being as effective functioning on its own. So give yourself a three-day break for your body to recover its peristaltic function.

Worried about caffeine withdrawal? Have some black tea! I love a good Darjeeling in the morning, and that contains almost as much caffeine as coffee. Enjoy a cup or two of black tea, which will also count toward your total water intake, but please don't have more than 2 cups a day, since that becomes more acid than your body wants.

Green tea may also be too acidic for you. I have seen it aggravate digestive issues and create acid reflux. Remember, hampered digestion can actually mean slowed weight loss. So for right now, let's play it safe and stick with herbal teas like peppermint or chamomile, or good old black tea.

Will you be the worst Metabolism Planner ever if you break down and have a cup of coffee on Day 2? Well, no. After all, you are still doing so many amazing things for your body! And you know what? The second time you do the cleanse—and, trust me, you will want to—you shouldn't have any issues with letting go of caffeine. This time around you are releasing decades' worth of toxins. Next time it will just be the toxins you accumulated over a few months. So do what you can, and that's all I can ask!

Can I Add Spices or Condiments?

Stay away from bottled condiments—that is, mustard, ketchup, barbecue sauce, chutney, and the like. While they are all great for livening up a dish, many of the ingredients may be inflammatory. Avoid them during your 30-day Metabolism Plan, and you can test them later.

If you have a sensitivity or an allergy to any spice or herb listed in your 30 days, please feel free to omit it. Below are anti-inflammatory spices and seasonings that are highly unlikely to trigger a reaction, so use as much of them as you like.

Spices to Enjoy
Basil
Black pepper
Cardamom
Cayenne
Chives
Cinnamon
Cloves
Cumin
Dill
Garlic
Ginger
Maine Sea Seasonings Kelp with Cayenne or Dulse (a blend of
    seaweed, which is great for an underfunctioning thyroid; do
    not use if you are hyperthyroid, though)

Nutmeg

Onion

Oregano

Rosemary

Sage

Thyme

Turmeric

You do want to avoid some potentially inflammatory spices until you get a chance to test them, particularly paprika, and especially mild paprika. You find it in a lot of prepared spice mixes, so keep an eye out!

Spices to Avoid

Chili powder

Fennel

Licorice

Paprika

Also avoid seasoning mixes that contain MSG, which triggers inflammation. Seasoning manufacturers are not required to disclose whether they include MSG, so steer clear of any spice mix that just says "spices" without listing the individual ingredients.

People often ask me whether they should include a spice that they already know is an issue for them. Please don't! Remember, if it's not healthy for you, then it's not healthy. If garlic, onions, or cayenne are allergens, please omit them and use another spice that you have tested and found to be friendly to your body.

The Ultimate Prep Tool: You

You have spent the last 10, 20, or 50 years trying to figure out what's going wrong and why your body isn't responding. I don't want you spending *one more day* on beating yourself up and asking "Why?" Dedicate the next 30 days to *you*. You are worth this investment of time and energy. I know you are going to rock this!

CHAPTER SEVEN

Days 1 to 3

The Cleanse

The next three days are a powerful introduction to what your body can do—and perhaps also a dramatic revelation of what you have been doing to your body! Best of all? In just three days, you experience a glorious change: weight loss, bright eyes, bright mood, brain as sharp as a tack—a total transformation.

I've been helping my clients do food-based cleanses for more than 25 years, and I can't think of a faster way to kick-start both healing and amazing weight loss. The foods you'll consume on the cleanse are nutrient-dense, chock-full of fiber, and loaded with protein. You're going to feel full and satisfied, yet at the same time, you're giving your body a break from digesting food that takes more energy to break down. And guess where that energy goes? Into deep repair, which in turn translates into weight loss. When my clients do the cleanse, the average weight loss for women is 5 pounds. For men, it's 7 or 8. I've even had some people lose 10 pounds in three days!

I'm so excited for you to have this fabulous experience of rejuvenation. It's the beginning of a whole new life.

Jeanine, Age 41

As a family practice physician, I was never taught about nutrition or counseling patients for weight loss. Every day I was confronted with patient after patient describing their frustration and confusion over how to lose weight, and I felt helpless. I tried to guide them, but every person had different results, or no results, and as soon as they stopped rigidly following the diet I gave them, they gained the weight back. I started to realize there was no one diet that fits every-one, because we are all unique.

Then I read a magazine article about Lyn-Genet. From a medical standpoint, her approach made total sense to me. I consider it the missing component in nutrition science. I met her in Houston and we started to work together right away. I am so happy I did this! I'm now at my goal weight. I feel amazing, I have more energy, I have no acid reflux symptoms, my gastrointestinal issues (bloating) are gone, and my sinus headaches are gone, too, as are the allergy pills. Best of all, my clothes fit again, and I don't have to buy a new wardrobe! Figuring out which foods I react to and cutting them out of my diet has transformed my health and my body.

I am thrilled to have another medical tool to help patients manage and even eliminate their chronic conditions such as migraines, arthritis, and depression. For the first time, some patients are discontinuing medications instead of adding new ones! This has been a life-changing experience, and I will never look at food the same way again.

The Detox Dilemma

I have devised the cleanse to be as easy for you as possible—no juice fasts or master cleanses here! Still, even during a gentle three-day cleanse, you might experience some discomfort from toxic buildup. Although some people sail through the detox, others develop some symptoms as a result of the poisons that are being released from fat cells—like environmental pollutants.

But look, it's better to get these toxins out of your body now, before they provoke serious disease. The good thing is that your body always wants to heal—really!—so if you give it a little help, it will work miracles for you. The symptoms won't last more than a few days, and it's better to deal with this now than later on when disease starts to crop up in a more serious form. I am here for you and know you will rock this!

Potential Detox Symptoms

Anxiety
Depression
Fatigue, lethargy
Gas
Headache
Indigestion
Irritability
Light-headedness
Loss of focus or concentration
Muscle aches

What Conditions Should Make You Cautious About The Metabolism Plan?

- **Diverticulosis and Crohn's disease**: The American diet is typically low in fiber, which creates a whole host of health problems—including diverticulosis and Crohn's disease. Unfortunately with diverticulosis, many people are still being told that they need to stick with a diet low in fiber. In fact, just the opposite is true: Only through higher-fiber diets can your body heal. However, you *do* need to avoid high fiber while you have *diverticulitis*, the active state of diverticulosis. Each person's tolerance to fiber is different, so I recommend that if you have a form of diverticulosis or

Crohn's, consult your health care provider before embarking on any major change to your diet, exercise regime or medication. I also recommend that you only do The Metabolism Plan under the care of a trained Metabolism Plan nutritionist. We start you off with a modified diet based on your current level of fiber intake to slowly reintroduce fiber into your diet so you won't have a flare-up.

- **Coumadin**: If you are taking a blood thinner that requires a diet low in vitamin K, download a custom menu from my website and have the diet approved by your doctor.
- **When pregnant and postpartum**: We do not recommend doing The Metabolism Plan when you are pregnant unless you are under the guidance of me or one of my staff; there are just too many variables to figure out! We have had many women successfully complete all 30 days of The Metabolism Plan when they are postpartum. However, if you find that the rapid weight loss is affecting your milk supply, please either discontinue or call my clinic to receive guided help.

The Pint Technique: How to Stay Hydrated

Make sure to drink your water *between* meals, not during meals, since that can impair digestion. If you can, leave a 45-minute window before and after each meal where you are not drinking water. Even more important: Finish the last of your water 45 minutes before dinner and do not consume any after dinner.

Now, I'm sure if you truly enjoyed drinking water, you would drink enough. But if you're like most people, you probably drink much less than you should. So if you don't like water, don't sip it all day. Knock it back all at once, a pint glass at a time!

For example, if you weigh 200 pounds, you need to drink six pints throughout the day. First thing in the morning, I want you to have one pint with lemon juice. Now you've got only five more pints to get through. Schedule one each at 9 a.m., 11 a.m., 2 p.m., 4 p.m., and 6 p.m.—and now you're done for the day.

Even better news? When you drink a pint all at once, your body takes what it needs and excretes the rest. So when you time your water intake, you can time your bathroom breaks, too.

Hydration Q&A

Q. What else can I drink besides water?

A. Most herbal teas are a terrific way to get in your water intake. Some recommendations are peppermint, chamomile, white, and rooibos teas. You may also have black tea, but I would limit it to 16 ounces daily because of its acidity. Avoid green tea completely, as it's even more acidic than black tea. While you are on The Metabolism Plan, I don't recommend teas that contain licorice, inulin, or chicory, because they usually slow weight loss. Wait to test them after your 30 days are over.

Q. Does coffee count as part of my water intake?

A. No, it doesn't. Once you've completed the cleanse, feel free to drink up to 16 ounces of coffee each day before or with breakfast.

Q. Do I need to drink extra water to compensate for coffee, tea, or caffeinated beverages?

A. No. But once you're through with the cleanse and are drinking wine again, please drink 4 extra ounces of water for every glass of wine.

Ready, Set, Cleanse!

So let's do a little checklist right now.

Have you been drinking your water based on your weight? Check! Done the yeast test? Check! Have all the supplements you need? Check! What about a high-quality scale and a good digital thermometer? Yes? Great! Now let's look at the shopping list for Days 1 to 3.

Spices and Herbs

Black pepper	
Cayenne	
Celery seed	*OPTIONAL*
Chipotle in adobo sauce or Sriracha sauce	1 jar
Cinnamon	
Cloves	
Cumin	
Ginger (fresh)	3 inches
Italian herb blend	
Low-sodium chicken broth (70 mg/cup)	1 container
Nutmeg	*OPTIONAL*
Olive oil	
Sea salt	
Turmeric	
Vanilla extract	

Nuts and Seeds

Almonds (raw and unsalted)	8 ounces
Chia seeds	Small bag
Flaxseeds	1 cup
Pumpkin seeds	8 ounces
Sunflower seeds	8 ounces

Fruits and Vegetables

Apples	3 apples
Avocados	1 avocado
Blueberries (fresh or frozen)	1 large container or 8- to 12-ounce bag
Cranberries (dried)	*OPTIONAL*
Lemons	4 lemons
Oranges	1 orange
Pears	1 pear
Beets	1 large beet
Broccoli	10 heads of broccoli
Carrots	5 pounds
Garlic	8 cloves

Herbs for a salad, such as basil or dill	Enough for three days' worth of salad
Kale	2 bunches
Lettuce—baby romaine	1 large container
Onions—red	5 large red onions
Shitake mushrooms	3 to 4 mushrooms
Zucchini	4 large zucchini
Raisins	1 small box

Miscellaneous

Basmati rice, uncooked	1 small bag
Brown sugar	A few spoonfuls
Coconut milk, full fat (canned)	2 8-ounce cans
Honey	1 jar
Silk Coconut beverage or Rice Dream	1 to 2 quart-sized cartons

General Guidelines for the Cleanse

- Follow the menus exactly. Do not make substitutions or changes.
- Salad dressing for the cleanse should consist of lemon juice, extra virgin olive oil, and whatever herbs you like (my own personal favorite is dill).
- Do not consume coffee during the cleanse. If you are concerned about a caffeine-withdrawal headache, you may have black tea. Green tea might aggravate acid reflux or worsen nausea, so please avoid it.
- Remember that all teas count toward your water intake. Please limit caffeinated teas to 16 ounces a day.
- Avoid all sweeteners during the cleanse, both the calorie and the no-calorie kind. And read the label even on your teas, because some teas contain stevia, chicory, licorice, or inulin, all of which might cause weight stabilization instead of weight loss.

Frequently Asked Questions About the Cleanse

Do I Have to Eat Everything Listed on a Particular Day?

The short answer is yes. Every single day, you're going to be eating a chemically balanced group of foods designed to achieve two goals: to give your body the nutrients it needs and to ensure you feel satisfied. Skipping part of a meal might mean missing out on protein, fat, fiber, or the nutrients that keep you full and primed for weight loss.

Will I Be Hungry?

I'll be honest with you: It's not very likely. You'll be eating nice, big portion sizes and getting all the nutrients you need. And at every meal, you're going to eat until you're full.

So if you do get hungry between meals, ask yourself: Did I *really* eat until I was full? Maybe, after years of dieting, you've gotten used to stopping yourself too soon.

The other possibility is that you've been skimping on your daily water intake. Dehydration is sneaky—it often masquerades as hunger—so when you think you need food, you might actually just need water.

The reason for this anatomical bait-and-switch is fascinating. Back when we were gatherers, plants were more plentiful than fresh running water. So ancient humans quenched their thirst with fruits and vegetables whose water content was high. In response, our brains create mixed signals, cuing us to crave food when what we really want is water.

Don't let your brain fool you! Make sure you're getting enough water before you reach for more food.

And if, after all that, you're *still* hungry? You can eat more veggies. Do not—repeat, do *not*—increase the portions of protein or fruit, which also means no extra nuts or seeds. Doing so could skew your overall sugars or protein for the day. Later on, you'll get to test portion sizes for proteins and fruits. For now, stick to the portions that we know won't trigger inflammation and weight gain.

What Will I Eat on the Cleanse?

ESSENTIAL EVOO

Extra virgin olive oil—a.k.a. "EVOO"—is one of my favorite fats. Not only is it delicious; it's some of the best brain food you could want. On The Metabolism Plan, you'll consume 3 to 5 tablespoons of EVOO a day. Why is EVOO so important? Well, your brain is 60 percent fat. If you don't replenish that fat, your brain goes hungry. Moreover, every one of our cells has a wall made of fat—technically, a *phospholipid* barrier. So we need fat to protect our cells and promote immune function.

Even better, EVOO is an omega-9, which acts as a catalyst for the anti-inflammatory properties of omega-3 (which on this program you will be getting from flaxseeds and chia seeds). Since inflammation packs on the pounds, you want to be loading up on foods that help you to bring it down.

Last but not least, fat keeps you feeling full longer! I don't want you hungry and miserable, and getting your daily serving of EVOO is a great way to prevent that.

I'll always remember the look on my client Gianna's face when she told me how excited she was about all the EVOO she could have on the Plan. "As an Italian I am embarrassed to say that I had given up olive oil because I thought it was fattening and raising my cholesterol," she told me. "I can't believe how delicious it is, how full I am, and how much weight I'm losing!" Of course, the icing on the cake was when she called me a month later to let me know her cholesterol had dropped more than 45 points!

Maria, Age 34

The Metabolism Plan has been a lifesaver! I was prediabetic, my cholesterol was 280, and my triglycerides were 215. I have lost 49 pounds so far; my cholesterol is 141; my triglycerides are 91; and my A1C [which measures blood sugars] is back in a healthy range. I feel good enough to exercise, which is so much easier now that my joints

---

no longer hurt. This doesn't even feel like a diet! We love the food. My husband has lost 91 pounds, his knee and back pain are gone, and he is playing soccer three times a week. I know this has saved both of us from a lifetime of medications.

THE LOWDOWN ON LETTUCE

When you look at the menus and meal plans on The Metabolism Plan, you'll see "baby romaine" as your daily lettuce choice. But if you can't find that, don't worry. There are plenty of other lettuces you can use. Boston lettuce, red and green leaf lettuces, frisée, escarole, and small amounts of radicchio are all terrific choices that will not disrupt thyroid function. If you want to try any other types of lettuces, however, you need to test them. Any mixed-greens blend that includes arugula, watercress, tatsoi, chard, raw kale, or spinach must be tested. Romaine hearts and iceberg lettuce often cause gas and bloating. In traditional Chinese medicine, all of these lettuces are known for being "cold" vegetables, renowned for slowing digestion. Remember, whenever you disrupt your digestion, you stall your weight loss.

FABULOUS FLAX

The Flax Granola on The Metabolism Plan is easy to make. You can bake it in big batches ahead of time. Or you can order it from my website (www.lygenet.com), and you will have it by the time you finish reading this book!

However you get it, our Flax Granola is rich in omega-3s, protein, calcium, and selenium. It also has mucilage, a gummy substance that has incredible benefits for your gastrointestinal tract and relieves constipation as well. Finally, flaxseed is extremely high in fiber, which supports colon detoxification, keeping you full and reducing sugar cravings.

After your first week on The Metabolism Plan, please limit your consumption of Flax Granola to twice a week if you want to get maximum health benefits. Remember, our motto is always "rotate or react," because even healthy foods can become unhealthy if you eat them too often. Don't worry—I'll be giving you plenty of other great tasty breakfast recipes as The Metabolism Plan continues.

Weekend Warriors

Most people like to shop on Friday after work, cook and prep on Saturday, and start their cleanse on Sunday. That way, you've got all your food ready so you can sail through your workweek. But as always, you should do what works best for *you*.

Each Day of the Cleanse

- Eat until you're full at every meal.

Even if you don't finish all the food, please make sure to have part of each recommended dish.

- Please remember to include EVOO, lemon juice, and herbs of choice as your lunchtime salad dressing.
- *Stay hydrated* by drinking half your body weight in ounces. Drink between meals—45 minutes away from eating. Try to finish all of your water 45 minutes before dinner and do not have any water after dinner for best weight loss.
- **Women**: When seeds or nuts are listed at any meal, please have 1 ounce.
- **Men**: When seeds or nuts are listed at any meal, please have 1.5 ounces.

Your Morning Routine

- Take your BBT (see page 45 for instructions).
- Weigh yourself and record the results in your journal.
- After weighing, drink 16 ounces of fresh water with lemon juice.
- Take supplements as needed.

DAY 1: LAUNCHING THE CLEANSE

If you start to feel detox symptoms, double-strength peppermint tea will often make them disappear. If aspirin is part of your protocol, feel free to take some if you feel a headache coming on. I find Excedrin Migraine and Bayer to be especially good. Try to avoid Advil and Motrin, as each pill can cause 0.2 to 0.4 pound of water retention per 200 mg. Avoid Tylenol— the products I recommend are better at not inhibiting weight loss.

Day 1 is a great time to schedule a little pampering to help your body in its restoration process. If you can, go for a short walk and do some gentle stretches. Hot baths or showers are great during the cleanse, especially on Day 1, as is 15 to 20 minutes in a sauna, which supports your organs of elimination.

Overall, your goal is to restore and nourish yourself, inside and out, so whether you make this a mini–spa day or a day watching football, make it a day that is all about *you*.

Detox Bath Salts

For a cleansing bath that pulls the toxins from your body, mix up some bath salts from the following recipe and soak for 20 to 30 minutes:

> 1 cup baking soda
> ½ lb Dead Sea salts
> 1 lb Epsom salts
> Essential oils of choice—or throw in a few herbal tea bags
>   such as sage or chamomile

BREAKFAST

Women: 1 cup Flax Granola (page 251) with ½ cup blueberries
Men: 1½ cups Flax Granola (page 251) with 1 cup blueberries
Served with Silk Coconut Milk or Rice Dream

LUNCH

Carrot Ginger Soup (page 252)

Women: 2 cups sautéed or steamed broccoli

Men: 3 cups sautéed or steamed broccoli

Baby romaine with fresh herbs of choice and sunflower seeds, dressed with EVOO, lemon juice, and herbs of choice

SNACK

1 medium-sized apple

DINNER

Kale with Spicy Coco Sauce (page 271) with sunflower seeds

Beet and Carrot Salad (page 257) with pumpkin seeds, lemon juice, EVOO, and your choice of herbs

DAY 2: TEST RAW ALMONDS

Day 2 incorporates your first test, which is almonds. It's essential that you choose raw, unsalted almonds since roasted nuts are more reactive. Early in The Metabolism Plan, we want to test as many vegetable and animal proteins as possible, so that we have the most possible choices for rotation. We deliberately start with the foods that most people can tolerate, so that you can quickly expand your list of friendly foods.

However, you might be in that small percentage of the population that has trouble with raw almonds. So if you find that you gain weight or are reactive to almonds in any way, please omit them from your menu going forward. There will be plenty of alternatives for you to choose from. Remember, you may be reacting badly only because you have been overdoing almonds or because of your general level of inflammation. So feel free to retest them in a few months, after you have given your body a break.

Now, how's the detox going? If you are feeling just awful, I have a trick! It will slow down the detox a wee bit, but I don't want you feeling rotten. Instead of having rice for dinner, switch it to lunch and omit the Carrot Ginger Soup. But keep the pumpkin seeds at dinner. This will make a huge difference in the way you feel, I promise!

BREAKFAST

Women: 1 cup Flax Granola (page 251) with ½ pear
Men: 1.5 cups Flax Granola (page 251) with 1 pear
Served with Silk Coconut Milk or Rice Dream

LUNCH

16 ounces Carrot Ginger Soup (page 252) with sunflower seeds
Baby romaine with ¼ avocado, EVOO, lemon juice, and herbs of
    choice (my favorite is dill!)
Women: 2 cups sautéed or steamed broccoli
Men: 3 cups sautéed or steamed broccoli

SNACK

Women: ½ apple and 8 to 10 almonds
Men: 1 apple and 16 to 20 almonds

DINNER

Kale with Spicy Coco Sauce (page 271)
1 cup basmati rice with pumpkin seeds
Beet and Carrot Salad (page 257) with sunflower seeds, lemon
    juice, and EVOO

DAY 3: TEST CHICKEN

Day 3 is a very mild test of chicken, an almost universally friendly protein. Remember, this first week we are stacking all the foods and exercise in your favor so you can lower inflammation while still gathering data. Chicken is a great protein to enjoy three or four times a week—just don't eat it two days in a row.

Enjoy today—you have worked really hard! Even if your detox symptoms are lingering, you're going to feel terrific really soon.

BREAKFAST

Women: 1 cup Flax Granola (page 251) with ½ apple
Men: 1.5 cups Flax Granola (page 251) with 1 apple
Served with Silk Coconut Milk or Rice Dream

LUNCH

Baby romaine with grated carrots, ¼ apple, and sunflower seeds,
    dressed with EVOO, lemon juice, and herbs
16 ounces Cream of Broccoli Soup (page 253)

SNACK

Spicy Roasted Pumpkin Seeds (page 267)

DINNER

Women: 2 to 3 ounces chicken, add approved herbs of your choice
Men: 4 to 6 ounces chicken, add approved herbs of your choice
Roasted Vegetables (page 256)
Baby romaine with ¼ avocado, EVOO, lemon juice, and herbs

Colleen, Age 37

A few years ago, I was diagnosed with ulcerative colitis. I ended up seeing a doctor who truly acted as though he wanted to help me. But the one thing he kept saying to me was, "This condition has never been shown to be affected by diet." And I believed him. I tried every prescription he could give me. Nothing worked. Life was miserable for me! He was about to put me on a steroid, but I was determined not to go that route.

Then I found out about Lyn-Genet. Because of my own experience with colitis and diet, the things I learned from her made sense to me. I ended up shedding 20 pounds. Now I sleep better, I have more energy, and my skin looks better. I didn't even realize how much bloat and swelling I was suffering from until it all went away. But far and away, the greatest change has been in my colitis. While I still have symptoms and flare-ups from time to time, I would say that I am 95 percent better!

Lyn-Genet has provided me with a relief that I never knew I could achieve. I can go jogging again without having to run laps around a restroom! I can sleep through the night without having to get up to use a restroom. If you don't have colitis, you will never understand how much these little things can mean!

Ending Your Cleanse

You did it! Your cleanse is officially over, and your body is so grateful you took this time to show it some love. Starting tomorrow, you'll begin the next phase of the program, in which you continue the testing process for food and start testing some baseline exercise. In this next phase, you'll begin to learn which kinds of movement your body loves while diversifying your diet with more delicious food.

- -

CHAPTER EIGHT

Days 4 to 10

Laying the Groundwork

Bravo! You've made it through the cleanse, and you're ready to move on to the next phase. This is where I like to say that life gets normal, so enjoy!

Every day I want this to be less *my* Metabolism Plan and more *your* Metabolism Plan. But to do that, we have to start testing your responses to different types of food and exercise so that you know exactly what works for you and what doesn't.

You know how you can go on a diet and it works for a little while and then it stops? That's because your chemistry changes! But when you know how the testing process works, you can keep adjusting your food and exercise as your body changes over the coming years, always making sure that your choices are the healthiest *for you.*

Sound good? Here's how we get started:

- On the even-numbered days, you test food.
- On the odd-numbered days, you test exercise.

On Days 5, 7, and 9, you are going to establish your baseline response to exercise. During this phase, the exercise is very mild. You might enjoy some mild weight loss, or that might not come until the next phase. You can expect to lose at least 0.5 pound each day, however, which is still a significant amount. Your ideal is a BBT of 97.0 to 97.3.

Our goal with exercise is not to overdo it, especially in the beginning, when we are setting up a successful framework—that's only going to create inflammation, a sluggish metabolism, and weight gain. On the other hand, I don't want you avoiding exercise because you think it's got to be all or nothing. You're going to learn your "sweet spot"—the amount and type of exercise that are just right for you.

What if you simply don't like exercise? Well, you may be like my son, Brayden, who says that his favorite sport is relaxing. It just so happens that with trial and error, I found a sport Bray loves and truly excels at—sprinting. Maybe that's because it's fast and he can get it over and done with quickly! I promise, there is an exercise out there that you, too, will enjoy, so let's get off that couch on Day 5 and find out exactly what your body wants and needs. Here comes the million-dollar trainer!

Cooking Hacks

- Pick a cooking day early in this phase and make your Cream of Broccoli Soup (page 253) and Lemon Basil Escarole Soup (page 254). All the soups freeze beautifully, by the way!
- Roast a chicken for the week or use the Crock-Pot recipe (page 272)—that's three or four dinners a week right there!
- Chop all of your vegetables—broccoli, yellow squash, onions, and kale—and store them. Make a batch or two of zucchini pasta. Or buy prechopped vegetables and zucchini pasta, which you can do in many stores. Do vegetables start to lose some nutrients this way? A little, but keeping stress levels down is important, too, so go ahead with some quick fixes as you start to find your own streamlined routines.

- Make a big batch of Trail Mix (page 267) and pre-measure out your portions as needed: ¼ cup for women, ½ cup for men.
- Buy Bare Apple Chips or use our recipe (page 269).
- On Day 6, you will test a new protein of your choice. One of the friendliest proteins is lamb. Like chicken, you can have lamb three times a week. Going forward, if lamb is friendly to you, I recommend buying big batches of ground lamb so you can make and freeze Lamb Burgers (page 273). With the recipe, I make burgers for me and my husband and lamb meatballs for the kids. It's so easy, and you can have weeks' worth of dinners frozen and ready when you need them!

What the Right Exercise Will Do for You

- Rev up your metabolism
- Balance your hormones
- Boost your mood
- Increase your energy levels
- Improve your quality of sleep
- Improve your muscle tone

Figuring Out the Puzzle

Remember our food reactivity chart (page 14)? There we saw some types of foods are more highly reactive, while other types of food are less reactive. Those numbers are for the general population, however—not necessarily for *you*. But I'm trying to stack the odds in your favor, so I'll always have you start with what works for most people. Once you've built up a list of friendly foods, you can methodically test more foods, always starting with those that are least likely to be reactive.

We are taking this same approach for exercise as well. Some types of exercise seem to work almost universally, while others are more likely to provoke an inflammatory reaction. So you'll start with the least reactive types and amounts of exercise, allowing us to establish your baseline response. We are looking for two things:

- the type and amount of exercise that produces better weight loss than you could get from just altering your diet alone
- the type and amount of exercise that helps your BBT reach the optimal range—the zone where your metabolism is performing at its peak.

Of course, many factors can lower your BBT, such as a lousy night's sleep or a rotten day at work. That's why if you have a negative reaction to a type and amount of exercise, we're going to test your response to that same type and amount two more times. If you still have a negative reaction after all three, your body probably doesn't like that exercise and would prefer another.

For example, suppose you're a runner, and you go for your 15-minute run. You'd expect to lose some weight and see your BBT bump up a little. But if you gain a pound and your BBT drops a full point, your body might be telling you that running is not for you, at least not right now, and you might want to think about testing a new exercise next week, or retest on your next test day.

You might be wondering why we test exercise three times but food only once during the 30 days. It's because your food response is based on your immune system, manifesting in weight gain and physiological symptoms, and the response to a food is much stronger than a response to exercise. Your exercise response is based on your thyroid (as measured by your BBT), which is more affected by such outside factors as sleep, stress, and hormonal fluctuations. If you find you test reactive to any food you love and are unsure of your data, you can always retest it.

Rotate or React

Suppose you pass your "running test" with flying colors. Then, on your next two test days that week, I suggest that you try out some other types of exercise and see whether your body likes them just as well, or even better.

"But I know what I like, and I passed the test—why can't I just stick with it?"

My clients ask me this all the time, and I'm going to tell you what I tell them: *Rotate or react.* You don't want to do the same type of exercise all the time, day after day, week after week. Changing up your exercise will help you achieve *optimal body composition*—that is, your ratio of lean muscle to body fat. Good body composition means you aren't just losing weight, but also improving how lean and toned you are. You have no idea how many people I work with are close to their goal weight but aren't happy with how they look when it comes to beach time. Aiming for your optimal body composition will fix that—promise!

Now, I know you might be a hard-core weight lifter and that's all you want to do, every workout for the rest of your life, but do me a favor. If you pass your first exercise, I want you think outside the box and try something new. C'mon, even pro football players practice ballet to improve their game! If one type of exercise passes the test, try another, and then another—you might be surprised to find out what your body likes! You might even switch up your exercise as the seasons change. Rotating both food and exercise keeps your body from reacting badly to something that might work well for you in small doses but is not healthy in larger doses.

My client Gregory discovered the benefits of switching exercise routines—although it wasn't exactly by choice. A longtime marathoner and lacrosse player, Gregory was highly successful at both sports throughout his 20s.

Then, in his late 30s, things started to change. He began to get injury after injury. The final straw came when he tore his ACL (the anterior cruciate ligament, a connective tissue in the knee—a common injury for lacrosse players). Gregory started rehab for his knee, but he was very upset about not being able to either run or play lacrosse. Angry and depressed, he resigned himself to swimming, a sport he had hated in his teens.

Then a surprising thing happened: Gregory started feeling terrific every time he left the pool. At first he thought it was just the endorphin rush that he would have gotten from any exercise. Eventually he realized his body actually loved swimming. His knee soon healed, but Gregory hung up his lacrosse stick and put away his running shoes. Two years later, swimming is still his sport of choice.

If Gregory could find joy in a new routine, you can, too. If you find out that your current exercise program is holding you back, you'll have a compelling reason to change it. And even if your body still loves what you're doing, it might love a little variety even more.

Choosing Your Exercise

The information we gather this week will lay the groundwork for the whole rest of the month. Here are the exercises that are the least inflammatory if you do them for less than 30 minutes:

Body-weighted exercise
Dancing
Pilates
Plyometrics
Running
Walking (if you are not used to walking)
Weight training
Yoga.

For the next few weeks, we'll avoid the following routines, which seem to have the potential to cause greater inflammation:

Boot camp
CrossFit

Heated yoga over 80 degrees
Spinning.

These types of cardiovascular exercises tend to be the least effective for weight loss and optimal body composition. In fact, Dr. Kenneth Cooper, the "godfather" of aerobic exercise, recanted on the benefits of excessive cardio after seeing so many of his peers pass away from diseases caused by oxidative stress such as heart disease and cancer. He now says that any aerobic exercise in excess of 20 minutes may be ineffective and may actually be harmful.

You should also avoid the following types of exercise, which just don't maximize your effort and can slow weight loss:

Elliptical
Exercise bike
Most cardio machines
Treadmill (honestly, outdoors is better, even for interval training)
Walking, for seasoned walkers.

So what gives with exercise machines? Research from the University of Tampa in 2013 stated that yes, initially you will have weight loss when starting to use a machine like a treadmill, but then your body adapts to the limited range of motion. Your metabolism adapts, too, and actually slows down.

Rather than plodding along on a treadmill or elliptical, the human body seems designed to burn more fat when you engage in short bursts. A quick dash away from a predator, followed by a brisk walk, and then another quick dash. A big effort to lift a weight, a bit of breathing room, and then another big effort. And to avoid the limited range of motion on virtually all machines, outdoors is better than on a machine.

So this week, we're going to test the types of exercise that your body is most likely to love—exercise that raises your heart rate gently, like walking, or that intersperses effort and rest, like the other types of exercise. We've got the best chance of getting your body to say *yes* to these types of exercise, so that is where we're going to start.

The Pros and Cons of Oxidative Stress

As we saw on page 94, oxidative stress is your body's natural response to the free radicals exercise produces. At the right level of oxidative stress, these free radicals trigger your body to make its own natural antioxidants, which is a *good* thing. Too much oxidative stress, however, and you get too many free radicals. That can lead to cell damage and a host of other problems.

One of your most important natural antioxidants is an enzyme called *super oxide dismutase (SOD)*. This is a powerful weapon against premature aging, free radical damage, and a host of other problems, including potential cardiovascular disorders. As we age, though, levels of SOD get lower, as most enzymes do. And guess what? When you don't exercise, your SOD levels also decrease—whereas when you exercise, they increase, protecting your body against oxidative stress and generally improving your health. So what you need to find is the level of exercise that increases SOD without overwhelming your body with more free radical damage than it can withstand. Luckily, your testing in the next 30 days is going to help you do just that.

Savvy About Sugar

I am often asked, "Which sweetener should I use?" Here's the list of approved sweeteners on The Metabolism Plan:

Agave
Honey
Maple syrup
Molasses
Sugar.

When I share this list with clients, it invariably leads to the incredulous response: "Sugar, are you sure you said that? Like, *white* sugar??"

The answer is yes. When you consume a nutrient-dense diet filled with proteins, fats, and fiber, a *little* sugar is not an issue.

Of course, if you were on a restricted diet of 1,200 calories—or even worse, 500 calories—a small amount of sugar would constitute a large part of your overall calories, and that *would* be a problem. But when you consume more than 2,000 calories a day in a diet that is rich in protein, fiber, fat, and nutrients, the 16 calories from a teaspoon of sugar just doesn't mean all that much.

Would another, less-processed sugar be a better choice? Probably, but if you spend every single second micromanaging minutiae like whether your sugar cane had a happy childhood and if you should switch to molasses, I think we have a bigger problem. Take care of the big picture and don't stress about every detail. That alone will add ten years to your life, trust me.

What I *do* care about are the non-glucose sugars, including products like aspartame and stevia. I want you to avoid those 100 percent—read on to find out why.

Avoid Aspartame

Like all the cells in your body, your brain cells rely on glucose—a form of sugar found in all carbohydrates—for their food. There is a wonderful part of your brain known as the blood-brain barrier, which keeps toxins from passing into your brain. However, glucose is allowed to pass through that barrier, allowing your brain to get its food.

Now, here's where it gets interesting. The molecular structure of aspartame is so similar to sugar that it, too, is allowed past the blood-brain barrier—and then it latches on to your brain cells. Your brain finds this very confusing, because the aspartame *feels* like glucose, but it doesn't actually provide any of the fuel your brain needs. So now your brain is desperate for some real glucose, and what's the best way to get it? Sweet, starchy foods with lots of refined sugars and carbs. So guess what aspartame makes you crave? Your brain wants its sugar fix, and it wants it *now*! Pretty soon you're knocking back a donut with your diet soda—and what do you think *that* does to your weight?

To make matters worse, artificial sweeteners cause water retention, which promotes further weight gain. But the worst part? Aspartame is linked to disorders like Alzheimer's and Parkinson's and multiple sclerosis. Not. Worth. It.

Skip the Stevia

My reluctance to give stevia the green light is based on what I've seen with thousands of people. When stevia is introduced into the diet, I see almost universal weight stabilization instead of weight loss. So do us both a favor and pass on the stevia.

Your Daily To-Do List

- Eat until you're full at every meal.
- Even if you don't finish all the food, please make sure to have part of each recommended dish.
- You are now free to have either lemon juice and EVOO, *or* either of the two vinaigrettes from the recipe chapter (page 265), on your salads.
- Stay hydrated by drinking half your body weight in ounces. Drink between meals—45 minutes away from eating. Try to finish all of your water 45 minutes before dinner and do not have any water after dinner.
- Soup portions are 16 ounces for women and 20 ounces for men. Please do not have more.
- **Women**: When seeds, nuts, or cheese is listed at any meal, please have 1 ounce. Animal protein portions are 4 to 6 ounces. Your egg portion is 3 eggs.
- **Men**: When seeds, nuts, or cheese is listed at any meal, please have 1.5 ounces. Animal protein portions are 6 to 8 ounces. Your egg portion is 4 eggs.

Your Morning Routine

- Take your BBT (see page 45 for instructions).
- Weigh yourself and record the results in your journal.
- After weighing, drink 16 ounces of fresh water with lemon juice.

- Take supplements as needed.
- Approved fruits for breakfast cereal on The Metabolism Plan are blueberries, pears, and apples.
  - **Women**: Half a piece of fruit or ½ cup of blueberries
  - **Men**: A whole piece of fruit or 1 cup of blueberries

DAY 4: TEST CHEESE

Aaaah, Day 4, when I am everyone's friend! You've experienced great weight loss on your first three days. That rapid loss indicates how high your inflammation levels were and how quickly they've subsided.

That's terrific—but we've still got further to go. I want you to keep losing weight and to do some major healing this week. So we're going to spend this week testing the least inflammatory foods and exercise. You should be losing a half pound every day, unless you introduce a food that doesn't work for *your* chemistry. If any food causes you to gain weight or not to lose it, take it out of rotation immediately. This allows your body to quickly overcome the inflammatory response and get rid of the extra weight. The good news? Now you know how your body responds to that food. No more "mystery" weight gain!

Here's some more good news:

- You may now have one large cup of coffee in the morning, with or before breakfast.
- Feel free to enjoy wine and chocolate below 65 percent cacao at night.

I know a lot of other diet experts encourage you to get chocolate with a higher cacao content. But here's what I have found—once you go higher than 65 percent, some of the compounds in chocolate can trigger inflammation and acid reflux...and that means weight stabilization or weight gain.

Meanwhile, hallelujah! You get to have coffee! There really aren't enough words to describe that delicious aroma, are there? That first time you smell it again, you think you have never smelled anything so fantastic. Enjoy that cup o' joe—you earned it.

Then, at lunch, your lips slowly touch the creamy, slightly salty goodness of goat cheese and your mouth explodes with flavor. When you get home that evening, you decompress with a deep sigh. If you love red wine, this is your magic moment. Enjoy.

But the love fest doesn't end there! Enjoy an ounce of your favorite chocolate after dinner, to top off your meal. Ahhhhhh. Life has never felt better.

BREAKFAST

> **Women**: 1 cup Flax Granola (page 251) with *one* of the following: ½ cup blueberries, ½ apple, or ½ pear—these are your friendly fruits
>
> **Men**: 1.5 cups Flax Granola (page 251) with *one* of the following: 1 cup blueberries, 1 apple, or 1 pear—these are your friendly fruits
>
> Served with Silk Coconut Milk or Rice Dream

LUNCH

> Leftover roasted vegetables, reheated and served on a bed of baby romaine with pumpkin seeds, along with hard or soft goat cheese

SNACK

> Carrots with raw almond butter
> **Women**: 2 tablespoons
> **Men**: 3 to 4 tablespoons
> OR
> Trail Mix (page 267)

DINNER

> Chicken with herbs or approved spices
> Baby romaine with carrots and ¼ avocado
> Zucchini Pasta (page 256) with Sunflower Pesto (page 262)

Which Are Better for Working Out—Free Weights or Machines?

There is less risk in machines, so they are pretty awesome if you are newer to working out or if you're recovering from an injury and want to safely increase the amount of weight you are lifting. The problem is that long term, machines target only the larger muscle groups, which creates muscular imbalance—and imbalance can lead to injury. You also need to use many different muscle groups in conjunction with each other to be fully functional—not a goal you can easily reach with machines.

By contrast, free weights use more muscle groups in addition to stabilizing muscles that work together in concert. This will make you stronger and more functional for everyday life, whether you are carrying groceries or shoveling snow. So machines are great for a specific amount of time and purpose. In the long run you're better off with free weights.

DAY 5: TEST EXERCISE

The scale will be interesting for you after your first test day. What if you failed goat cheese? Well, first of all, I recommend that you retest it at some point. You can do that starting on Day 21, when you begin to make your own menus. And if it doesn't work for now and you need a dairy-free menu, you can download one from my website. Either way, you are now going to test exercise at the least reactive amounts possible—meaning there's no way you can fail this and we are now establishing your baseline response to exercise.

I want you to take whatever exercise routine you have been doing and start with the time frames listed on the following page. Not sure what you would like to do? Pop on over to my website and try out some of our free videos! And, dear folks who have been enjoying a guilt-free break from exercise, we're not asking you to do much, so don't worry!

So here are your guidelines for exercise for Days 5, 7, and 9.

Beginner: 4 to 6 minutes
Intermediate: 8 to 12 minutes
Advanced: 15 minutes

New to exercise and feeling a little overwhelmed? Here is a great beginner's routine, which is also on my website. You can do each exercise for 30 to 45 seconds, taking breaks as indicated if you need them. This routine will work your legs, glutes, hamstrings, shoulders, abs, pecs, back, and arms. It will also improve cardiovascular function. If you have knee or hip issues, always choose the low-impact (LI) option when you're given that choice.

1. Squats (LI)

Stand with your head facing forward, your chest held up, and your feet hip width apart.

Sit back as though you are trying to sit in a chair, keeping your chest and gaze facing forward. This will prevent your low back from rounding, which can cause lower back pain.

Lower down so your thighs are parallel with the floor. Don't let your knees come too far forward.

Come back up to standing position.

Repeat until the time is up, increasing your speed as you feel more comfortable.

2. Jumping Jacks, Jump Rope, or Marching (LI) or Jogging in Place

It's your choice here—time to get back to your playground favorites! Jumping jacks have the advantage of warming up your shoulder girdle.

3. Toe-Touch Kicks (LI)

Stand with your feet hip width apart and your hands reaching overhead. Do a high forward kick with your right leg, bringing your left hand to meet your toes. Repeat with the left leg and the right hand touching the toes.

4. *Lunges (LI)*

Stand with your feet together. Step your right foot forward as far as possible but don't let your knee come too far over your ankle, to prevent knee injury. Step your right foot back and repeat the sequence with your left foot. As you feel comfortable, build up speed.

Take a break here if you need to decrease your heart rate.

5. *Downward Dog (LI)*

Get down onto your hands and knees. Make sure your wrists are directly beneath your shoulders and your knees are directly below your hips.

Extend your elbows, keeping your back relaxed.

Spread your fingers out so that you can distribute your weight evenly throughout your hands, which will be supporting your weight.

Exhale as you tuck your toes, pressing through your feet and hands to lift your knees off the floor, so that your weight is supported by your hands and feet. Shift your pelvis up into the air, and then pull your sit bones down to face the wall behind you, so your whole body makes an upside-down "V." Keep your body extended—don't walk your feet or hands closer to each other.

Rotate your arms outward so that the creases in your elbows face your thumbs.

Pull your chest in toward your thighs so that you lengthen your spine.

Pull your thighs inward while lifting up your sit bones and pulling your heels down toward the floor.

Line up your ears with your upper arms, keeping your head relaxed but not hanging. Look back at your navel or between your legs.

Hold for 30 to 45 seconds.

To release, exhale while bending your knees so that you come back down to your hands and knees.

6. Push-ups (LI)

You can choose either a modified or full push-up. Get in a plank position with your legs fully extended in back of you, or, for the modified position, with your knees on the ground.

Slowly bend your elbows halfway as you draw your shoulder blades together.

Come back up to plank position. Repeat.

7. Crunches (LI)

Lie on your back with your knees bent. Clasp your hands gently behind your head.

Lift your torso as high as you can without your lower back leaving the floor. Think of keeping your nose in alignment with the ceiling.

Release down.

Repeat.

DAY 5 MENU

BREAKFAST

TMP Smoothie (page 248)

LUNCH

Baby romaine with radicchio, grated raw beet, and pumpkin
  seeds
Cream of Broccoli Soup (page 253)

SNACK

Carrots with raw almond butter
  • **Women**: 2 tablespoons
  • **Men**: 3 to 4 tablespoons
OR
Bare brand Apple Chips OR Apple Chips (page 269)

DINNER

Chicken with Spicy Apricot Glaze (page 263)
Sautéed zucchini with onion, basil, lemon juice, and ½ ounce
  Manchego
Baby romaine with pomegranate

Why Is My BBT So Low?

We are so early on in your exercise regimen that we shouldn't see a huge change in your BBT, but keep this in mind for going forward: The wrong type or amount of exercise for your body will cause your BBT to drop. But there are many other factors that might drive it down as well, particularly stress.

When you're having a rough day or week, your body is in a near-constant state of alertness to deal with the next stressor. Here are a few quick solutions to break out of this cycle:

- **SAM-e**: A miracle supplement whose effects you can feel within the hour. Most people do well with 600 mg taken all at once.
- **Meditation**: Just a few minutes at the beginning or end of your day can lower your stress hormones and get your relaxation hormones flowing. You can check the Resources for links to some websites that will get you started.
- **Lemon balm**: Taken as an extract, tea, or capsule (see page 62); or hops (see page 63).
- **Fun and joy**: Whether it's laughing at your favorite movie or hopping on the phone with a good friend.
- **Increased sleep**: Skimping on sleep drives your BBT down, which can affect your weight. I recommend an "electronic sundown"—no screens for two hours before you go to bed, since the flickering blue light behind the screen fools your brain into thinking it should be awake. Some bedtime meditation can also help calm you into sleep. Lemon balm and hops (see pages 62 and 63) are both good natural sleep aids and work well when taken at 5 p.m. or so.

- **Hormones**: Ladies, your BBT will rise when you ovulate, and again five to seven days before your cycle. It will drop once your cycle starts. I want you to use the higher numbers as your baseline numbers. Note that you may be more reactive during these times, so you might stay only with foods and exercises that you have already found friendly.
- **Vegetarian days**: Going meatless and fishless can sometimes deprive you of essential nutrients that your brain needs to organize sleep. The solution is to find optimal proteins that can offset this effect, and perhaps to take B12 to boost your thyroid function.
- **Being cold**: There's nothing better for sleep than a slightly cool room and a warm bed. But if you're sleeping *too* cold, your thyroid is working harder than it should. Try some cozy pajamas or a slightly warmer room. Drinking warm teas instead of cold water during the day can help, too.

DAY 6: TEST A NEW PROTEIN

Good morning! Yesterday was a big day! You are on the road to finding out how your body responds to exercise. What can you do on your off exercise days? Whatever your body doesn't perceive as stress; you can use your BBT to see what your body likes best. Gentle movements that don't increase heart rate work for just about everyone! For most people it is an easy 10- to 15-minute walk, 10 to 15 minutes of gentle yoga or stretching, or 5 minutes of abs.

Today, you are going to test one of the least reactive proteins. Here are your choices, with portion sizes listed on page 166:

- Beef
- Lamb
- Wild whitefish, preferably halibut or flounder
- Duck breast
- Eggs.

If you choose eggs, please make sure to follow these guidelines.

- **Women**: Use 3 eggs with kale or broccoli.
- **Men**: Use 4 eggs with kale or broccoli.

Rotate or React: The Protein Story

Throughout your 30 days, you're going to test a wide variety of proteins. You might discover that at this point, your body just doesn't like some of them, so you'll avoid those proteins for now. In three months to a year, you might retest the ones that didn't work, and you may be able to bring them back into your diet. Your body keeps changing, so foods that don't work now might work later, especially as you keep reducing inflammation and improving digestion.

But what about the proteins your body *does* like? Here's where the principle of "rotate or react" becomes so very important. A protein that works quite well for you after just one day might trigger inflammation if you consume it many days in a row. And some proteins are easier to tolerate than others. So once you know which proteins work for you, I want you to rotate them according to the following plan.

> **Chicken**: 3 to 4 times a week, every other day
> **Beans**: 3 to 4 times a week, every other day
> **Lamb**: 3 times a week, every other day
> **Duck breast**: 3 times a week, every other day
> **Eggs**: 3 times a week, every other day
> **Pork**: 1 to 2 times a week, several days apart
> **Turkey**: 1 to 2 times a week, several days apart
> **Fish and seafood**: 2 times a week, several days apart
> **Venison**: 1 to 2 times a week, several days apart
> **Beef**: 1 time a week
> **Bison**: 1 time a week

If you consume any of these proteins more often, they tend to become inflammatory. Remember, inflammation can cause diseases like heart disease and cancer. So yes, if you eat red meat five times a week, I could definitely see an increased risk for disease! In moderation, most people do marvelously with it.

BREAKFAST

Flax Granola (page 251) with friendly fruit of choice
Served with Silk Coconut Milk or Rice Dream
OR
Blueberry Compote (page 249)

LUNCH

Baby romaine with leftover zucchini, ¼ avocado, pumpkin seeds, and Manchego
Lemon Basil Escarole Soup (page 254)

SNACK

1 ounce Bare Apple Chips OR Apple Chips (page 269)
OR
Trail Mix (page 267)

DINNER

Your choice of grilled steak, lamb, wild whitefish (preferably halibut or flounder), or duck breast; OR eggs with kale and broccoli (portion sizes are on page 166)
Roasted Vegetables (page 256)
Baby romaine with ¼ avocado and herbs of choice

Jeremy, Age 38

Twenty years ago, I started running daily to lose weight, and back then, it really worked. About three years ago, I started having some injuries, and my cholesterol and weight started to pile on.

Based on the principles of The Metabolism Plan, I decided to switch up my exercise a bit to prevent injuries and lose weight. I started biking in the summer, and swimming and doing yoga in the winter. That was just what I needed to get both my weight and my cholesterol to go down, while my energy went up.

So far, I have lost 25 pounds just by eating foods that worked for me. I found out I liked both biking and swimming so much that I did my first triathlon this year. It was great to see my daughters cheering Daddy on. They felt so proud of me, but what really made me happy was that I feel I am setting such a great example for them.

Type II Muscle Fibers: Your Secret Weight-Loss Weapon

If you haven't tried sprinting or plyometrics in a while, consider it now. My long runs are history for now, but in the meantime, my body loves sprinting. I find this is true for a lot of my folks who found that long runs were no longer working for them.

Sprinting and plyometrics involve type II muscle fibers, your secret weight-loss weapon. The type I fibers are known as "slow twitch" muscles, and they seem to work better for distance running. Basically, they have gotten very good at using oxygen for fuel to support extended activity, like a marathon or a bicycle race. By contrast, type II fibers, known as "fast twitch," are more for the "get in and get out" type of exercise. Rather than using oxygen to create fuel—the so-called *aerobic* pathways—they use a different type of pathway, known as *anaerobic.*

Here's where the weight loss comes in, because anaerobic pathways are better at burning body fat. In fact, once you kick off this fat-burning effect, it continues long after you're actually done exercising. If you do enough anaerobic exercise, the fat burning is basically continuous, which means that you're losing body fat even when you're watching TV or talking on the phone. Not bad!

Now you see why we're looking for "bursting" type exercises—movement that requires short bursts of intense energy, rather than sustained exertion. The short bursts build type II muscle fibers, rely on anaerobic pathways, and lead to fat burning, all of which are terrific both for overall weight loss and for body composition.

DAY 7: TEST OR RETEST EXERCISE

Yesterday was a big day—I hope you passed your first protein test! Did you know that for optimal weight loss, you want to be able to rotate at least three proteins? This not only gives you a wide array of nutrients, but also makes it less likely that you will build up a food sensitivity that can turn into a food allergy.

There is no food test today, because we are going to focus on exercise. If your last test showed up negative—if you gained weight or had a suboptimal BBT, you can retest the same exercise because your data might have been affected by stress, sleep issues, or other factors.

If your previous type of exercise did pass, I would love it if you tried a new type of exercise today. Remember, your goal is to have several different types of exercise that work for you so that you can support your body in a wide variety of ways. However, if you are brand-new to exercise or haven't worked out in a while, feel free to stick to the routine I gave you on page 170, or try one of the videos on my website (www.lyngenet.com).

Beginner: 4 to 6 minutes
Intermediate: 8 to 12 minutes
Advanced: 15 minutes

BREAKFAST

Flax Granola (page 251) with friendly fruit of choice
Served with Silk Coconut Milk or Rice Dream
OR
Apple Streusel (page 249)

LUNCH

Leftover roasted vegetables, reheated and served on a bed of
baby romaine with almond slivers

Cream of Broccoli Soup (page 253)

SNACK

1 ounce salt-free potato chips with Zucchini Noush (page 269)

OR

Trail Mix (page 267)

DINNER

Chicken with herbs of choice or approved spices (page 139)

Sautéed vegetables: Broccoli, yellow squash, and scallions

Baby romaine and grated carrots and herbs of choice

DAY 8: TEST A NEW PROTEIN

Today you get to take your third protein test. I am rooting for the
foods you love to pass! I also want you to develop an arsenal of food
choices as quickly as possible so you can start to rotate them.

BREAKFAST

TMP Smoothie (page 248)

LUNCH

Leftover sautéed vegetables on a bed of baby romaine with
Chicken Kale Soup (page 254)

SNACK

Trail Mix (page 267)

OR

Spicy Roasted Pumpkin Seeds (page 267)

DINNER

Test a new protein—beef, lamb, wild whitefish, duck breast, or
eggs. If you choose eggs, see page 166 for portion sizes, and
add broccoli and kale.

Zucchini Pasta (page 256) sautéed with scallions and topped with
grated Manchego

Baby romaine with grated carrot and herbs of choice

DAY 9: TEST EXERCISE

Today is your last day for testing basic exercise. Next week, we're
going to step it up a bit, but for now, we're still checking out the
friendliest possible workouts. If there is any exercise you are unsure
of, please retest it today.

If your Day 7 test was successful, consider trying something
new—perhaps that schoolyard favorite, jumping rope? Did you know
it's a great warmup or complete workout? Jumping rope is not only
great for getting your heart rate up, but also fantastic for building the
muscles in your biceps, forearms, and shoulders. If your knees and
ankles can tolerate a high-impact workout, enjoy some schoolyard
fun! This in conjunction with planks and pushups is a great at-home
workout.

Because we're testing exercise today, we're going to focus on
foods that we already know your body likes. Remember, you only
ever want to test one thing a day—just one new food or one new
thing about your exercise—so that the next day, you know exactly
what your data means.

Beginner: 4 to 6 minutes
Intermediate: 8 to 12 minutes
Advanced: 15 minutes

BREAKFAST

Flax Granola (page 251) with friendly fruit of choice
Served with Silk Coconut Milk or Rice Dream

LUNCH

Sautéed kale with TMP Caesar dressing (page 266), avocado,
apple, and pumpkin seeds
Lemon Basil Escarole Soup (page 254) or Carrot Ginger Soup
(page 252)

SNACK

Low-sodium potato chips (1 ounce)
OR
Trail Mix (page 267)

DINNER

Any friendly protein (to help you choose, see "Rotate or React:
The Protein Story" on page 175; portion sizes on page 166)
Leftover roasted vegetables
Baby romaine with grated carrots and herbs of choice

Hannah, Age 56

I was always the chubby kid, so my mom had my thyroid tested when I was a teen. My doctor put me on Synthroid, and I resigned myself to always being the "friend on a perpetual diet."

Then I found out my coworker had done The Metabolism Plan and was able to cut her thyroid meds in three weeks. I was so surprised! I thought once you were on them that was it for life. Maybe there was hope for me.

Sure enough, I started The Metabolism Plan and wasn't allowed to exercise for the first four days. I was shocked when I lost 7 pounds in four days! That would normally take two months if I counted every calorie. When I found out that I only needed to exercise eight minutes to see results, that was my idea of heaven, and sure enough I kept losing weight. I've lost 24 pounds in two months and have been able to cut my meds by 50 percent. My mom is so thrilled with my results that she started The Metabolism Plan too. Now she is off her blood pressure meds and her arthritis is better!

DAY 10: TEST A NEW PROTEIN

Here's an extra day to establish a new protein that works for you. We want you rotating your proteins—but to do that, you've got to have as many proteins as possible in your arsenal.

Keep in mind, your body might be ready for a change. If you've been eating lots of red meat, your body might be longing for something new and will respond beautifully when you test fish and eggs. If you've been on more of a vegetarian diet, your body might have maxed out on beans and grains and may need some new proteins.

There's a reason we say "rotate or react": Your friendly foods are based on your nutritional needs—and those needs are always in flux! The great thing about The Metabolism Plan is that you don't get locked into any patterns after they've stopped working for your body. Your trusty scale and digital thermometer let you know right away what your body does and does not like.

BREAKFAST

Flax Granola (page 251) with approved fruit of choice (see page 168)
Served with Silk Coconut Milk or Rice Dream

LUNCH

Cream of Broccoli Soup (page 253)
Baby romaine with almond slivers and carrots

SNACK

> Spicy Roasted Pumpkin Seeds (page 267)
> OR
> Trail Mix (page 267)

DINNER

> Your choice of a new protein: grilled steak, lamb, wild whitefish
>   (preferably halibut or flounder), duck breast, venison, scallops,
>   lentils, tempeh, or pinto beans on a bed of romaine; OR eggs,
>   cooked any style, with kale, yellow squash, and broccoli
> Sautéed kale with scallions and grated Manchego

Franne, Age 29

I lost 13 pounds in 20 days! I am officially shocked! I consistently lost weight with 30- to 40-minute runs and *gained* weight with my 75-minute runs. Well, guess who has more time to sleep in? And as Lyn-Genet says, sleep aids weight loss. Thanks to her great tips and practical everyday advice, I am now weight training instead of running one or two days each week. I look more toned and can actually run faster! The Metabolism Plan rocks!

Tips from the Experts: Andia Winslow, Professional Athlete and Master Certified Fitness Professional

Tips for Newbies or Those Returning to Exercise

Many folks psych themselves out before their workout regimen even begins. The "I'm not ready yet" or "I have to get fit before I can go to the gym" mentality is the biggest saboteur that I've encountered in my professional experience. Conversely, other folks jump out of the gates too hard and fast. In an attempt to make up for lost time or to make quick gains, they overdo it and often injure themselves, which lands them back on the sidelines.

If you find yourself doing either, remind yourself to take it one day at a time, one gain at a time. Your goal is to design a program that is manageable and sustainable. You also want to change things up every three to four weeks to ensure that your body does not become too accustomed to the work and plateau.

Moving Forward

By now you're seeing how quickly you can heal, how much weight you can lose, and how you are able to get stronger after just a few days of exercise. You've done a great job at laying some solid groundwork that you can keep building on. Get ready to gather some more incredible data during Days 11 to 20, so that you can be at 110 percent every day!

CHAPTER NINE

Days 11 to 20

Stepping It Up

Now that you've finished Laying the Groundwork, you're ready to start Stepping It Up. This is one of the most exciting phases in your Metabolism Plan, because you get to greatly expand the number of foods you test. That gives you two big advantages: You learn which foods don't work for you, so you can avoid them, and you learn which foods your body loves, so you've got more friendly choices to rotate.

You get to ramp up your exercise, too. Either you'll stick with the same types you did last week and step up the duration and/or intensity (doing the same exercise longer, faster, or with more weight), or you'll test some new forms of exercise at the same duration and intensity you were at last week.

Suppose last week you tested jogging and weight lifting. On Days 4 to 10, you might have jogged for 12 minutes and done reps while lifting 25 pounds of weight. So now your Days 11 to 20 might look like this.

Day 11: Jog 15 minutes (20 percent increase in time from last week).

Day 12: Rest (and test a new food!).

Day 13: Lift 30 pounds (20 percent increase in weight from last week).

Day 14: Rest (and test a new food!).

Day 15: Jog 15 minutes (20 percent increase in time from last week).

Day 16: Rest (and test a new food!).

Day 17: Lift 30 pounds (20 percent increase from last week).

Day 18: Rest (and test a new food!).

Day 19: Your choice of jogging or lifting; or, combine jogging *and* lifting—say, jog for 10 minutes and lift 30 pounds for 5 minutes—and test that.

Day 20: Rest (and test a new food!).

Remember: You test exercise on odd-numbered days and food on even-numbered days. On the days when you test exercise, you eat only foods that you have already tested and know to be friendly. On the days when you test food, you take a break from exercise. If you test a new food and a new level of exercise on the same day, and you gain weight, you won't know which factor your body is reacting to.

Cooking Hacks for Days 11 to 20

- Pick a cooking day early in this phase and make your Chicken Kale Soup (page 254), Cream of Broccoli Soup (page 253), and, if you choose, the optional Lemon Basil Escarole Soup (254). Remember, all the soups freeze beautifully, so you can make them ahead of time and store for when you need them.

- Roast a chicken for the week or use the Crock-Pot recipe (page 272)—now you've got three or four dinners ready to go!

- Chop all of your vegetables—broccoli, yellow squash, onions, and kale—and store in the containers of your choice. Or buy prechopped vegetables, which you can do in many stores. Again, don't worry about whether the vegetables lose a few nutrients—you will more than make it up by the stress you save in streamlining your routine!

- Make zucchini pasta. Now that this is becoming second nature, you might want to get your kids involved—they will love using the spiralizer! We want to start getting the whole family on board with this way of eating.
- Make a big batch of Trail Mix (page 267) and measure out your portions as needed: ¼ cup for women, ½ cup for men.
- Tired of cooking? See if you can get a Chinese restaurant to make you plain steamed proteins—the ones you know are friendly— and some Metabolism Plan–friendly vegetables. Then add your own sauces from the recipe section (the Mango Salsa, page 262, is great for this). Make sure to tell them to leave out all salt, soy sauce, and MSG—just steam everything plain, with no seasoning. You can also order in. Make one day a test of sashimi, have some leftover vegetables, and take a night off!

Finding the Right Fitness Goals: Working Smarter, Not Harder

Often we get so stuck in the here and now, we start chasing goals that sound good but don't really serve us. We look for statistics to verify our progress—evidence that we're working harder—while forgetting that fitness is supposed to last a lifetime. Our ultimate goal is not to rack up numbers on a chart, but rather to remain strong, lean, and energized.

To this end, I'm going to help you find the fitness objectives that are perfect for *you*. Here are some of my favorite goals to keep you injury-free while preventing your routines from becoming ho-hum.

Fitness Goal 1: Be in it for the long run

Which is better: a super-demanding routine that you can sustain for only a few weeks, or a routine that fits easily into your lifestyle? I'll give you a hint: You want the routine that doesn't stress you out or make you feel as though you don't have enough time to do the other things you enjoy.

One glance at any child will tell you how much pure joy you can find simply in moving your body. Remember how much fun you had during recess and playing at the park? When you were a teenager, did you like to go dancing? Your body was made to move, and it craves movement. But if you haven't moved for a while, you kind of forget the fun.

You want a wide range of activities available, so that if one type creates inflammation or just becomes boring, you've got lots of other choices ready to go. Some of you will be doing triathlons in your 70s. Others will be happier doing yoga or tai chi. Whatever your goals, you want a wide variety of options that fit your needs at every stage of your life.

Karen, Age 39

For years, I kept thinking, "What's wrong with me? Why does everyone else have it so easy? Why am I such a loser?" I worked my butt off trying to do everything right, and I exercised to death, yet kept gaining weight.

Then I ran into an old workout friend who had lost 50 pounds over a year exercising 20 minutes every other day! When she told me what she was doing, I almost fell off my chair. But the more she talked, the more it made sense. So I started working with Lyn-Genet, and all of a sudden I knew everything was going to be okay. And it was. Like my friend, I had to cut way back on exercise to see results and eat way more to stop my body from thinking it was "famine time."

Now I've got my life back. I can eat out with friends, I'm not killing myself at the gym, and I feel good about me. My body doesn't feel like the enemy anymore.

Fitness Goal 2: Maintain flexibility

Most people lose flexibility and balance as they age, but that doesn't have to happen to you. Decreased flexibility can lead to injuries and arthritis. Decreased balance can increase your risk of falling, especially as you get older. Not the kind of old age I want for you!

How do you stay flexible? Always include some sort of stretching in your workout routine. In the short run, you'll get long and strong muscles. In the long run, you'll prevent injury. Win-win!

Brad, Age 42

I developed an autoimmune disease at the age of 40. I think it was mostly my high-stress job and crappy eating, but who knows? All I did know was that I loved my long bike rides. Riding 50 or 100 miles or even more on the weekend and doing the loop around Central Park kept me sane. Or so I thought. So I totally freaked out when Lyn-Genet said I couldn't do my rides the first two weeks on her program. She said that my system was so depleted, this level of exercise was just too stressful for me. I was beyond upset. But really, at that point I was starting to be so exhausted I secretly welcomed the break.

So I started The Metabolism Plan. Every day I took my BBT and did a little exercise—just a little. Within days my energy came back in droves and my BBT started to rise. All of a sudden I was thinking clearly and felt at the top of my game. I was sleeping through the night and started to feel less stressed.

Then Lyn-Genet said I could restart the bike rides, but she wanted me to test them. I was shocked—I failed. In every possible way: BBT down, weight up, energy down, symptoms up. We tested them three different times, but each time, we got the same results. I was so bummed.

So Lyn-Genet helped me focus on different fitness goals. She recommended plyometrics, sprints, and kettlebells, and I have to say I'm really enjoying these new routines. They have the intensity that I like, but the shorter bursts of energy and time work better for my immune system.

Now my autoimmune symptoms are in remission and life is good. Thanks to The Metabolism Plan, I feel like I've got another 50 years of training and exploring to do.

Fitness Goal 3: Lower your body fat percentage

So often I hear people talk about weight. But what the scale says—as helpful as it may be—can also be such an arbitrary number. After all, 130 pounds with 30 percent body fat looks very different from 130 pounds with 20 percent body fat!

I'm sure you have heard that old myth that a pound of muscle weighs more than a pound of fat? That one drives me crazy—a pound is a pound is a pound! However, it *is* true that a pound of muscle takes up less space than a pound of fat, so you look leaner with better muscle tone. Plus, the more muscle you have, the more metabolically active you are. Even when you're sitting on the couch or lying in bed, your muscles keep your metabolism humming, so that a greater percentage of muscle helps *keep* you thinner. Less fat and more muscle means better weight loss.

Want to know your body fat percentage? You can talk to a trainer at the gym and have them measure you once a month, or you can buy a handheld body fat monitor. I use Omron (see Resources). If you already have a scale with body fat percentages, please be cautious about the data, because I find this type of scale to be pretty inaccurate.

Fitness Goal 4: Get stronger

Strength is an important goal for many reasons. Physically, it means you're building bigger, stronger muscles, and as we just saw, that's great for your weight, your metabolism, and your health. But strength also makes you feel terrific. You can lift a suitcase, tote boxes out to the garage, give a horsy ride to a young child—so many activities that make you feel strong and powerful.

So I encourage you to set new strength goals. Get creative and come up with objectives that fit your own personal interests and workout routine. Maybe you're currently doing 10 push-ups and you want to get up to 25. Maybe you're running a 10-minute mile and you want to bring it down to 8. Extend the number of reps you do or the amount of time you can work out. Whatever you decide, set goals that involve challenging your muscles.

Fitness Goal 5: Master a skill

Not really thrilled with running or lifting weights? Think the gym is just a ho-hum experience? Try piquing your interest by mastering a new skill, whether it's doing a handstand, learning how to box, or trying out a totally new sport like volleyball. A great side benefit to learning new skills is that they can also improve brain function!

Goitrogens: The "Healthy" Foods That Hurt Your Thyroid

A *goitrogen* is a food that depletes thyroid function. You don't necessarily need to avoid all goitrogens, but I don't want you eating them every day, either. Here are the foods you should test and some guidelines on how often to eat them.

Most Common Goitrogens

- Asparagus
- Barley
- Bok choy
- Broccoli (raw only)
- Broccolini—gai lan
- Broccoli rabe
- Brussels sprouts
- Cabbage
- Cauliflower
- Collard greens
- Edamame
- Kale (raw only)
- Mustard
- Mustard greens
- Nectarines
- Peaches
- Peanuts
- Pine nuts

- Radishes
- Raspberries
- Soy of all types, including tofu, miso soup, and soy-based proteins
- Spinach
- Strawberries
- Sweet potatoes
- Swiss chard
- Turnips
- Walnuts
- Watercress
- Wasabi

Can other foods be goitrogens? Absolutely! You will sometimes see lists that include wheat, rye, millet, and other grains. However, *any* reactive food can lower your BBT. That doesn't necessarily make it a goitrogen. You may find other lists in other sources, but this is my list based on what I have seen after working with thousands of people in my clinical practice.

A good rule of thumb is to test each goitrogen because, again, it might not be a goitrogen *for you*. If it does depress your BBT, skip it for now. You can always retest it in six to twelve months.

What about the goitrogens that pass your test? Limit each individual goitrogen to once a week and follow these guidelines.

- **If you have no thyroid issues or are hypothyroid (underactive thyroid):** If you don't have a thyroid issue, you don't want to develop one! And if you are hypothyroid, you want to give your thyroid a break. So, either way, consume at most three goitrogens per week, never two days in a row, and make sure they are three different goitrogens. For example,
  Monday: Strawberries
  Wednesday: Spinach
  Saturday: Brussels sprouts.

- **If you are hyperthyroid (overactive thyroid):** Aim for 4 to 5 goitrogens per week, spaced out throughout the week, but make sure they are different goitrogens. This can actually help bring down your thyroid function to a healthy level. For example,
Monday: Strawberries
Tuesday: Spinach
Thursday: Peanut butter
Friday: Swiss chard.

The important thing with goitrogens is to *test them* and then to *rotate them*. My client Janet learned this the hard way.

Janet was hypothyroid, and she really loved peanut butter. I mean *really*. So she kept pushing to test her beloved peanut butter. When she tried it, her BBT did not drop, and she lost only 0.2 pound—not the 0.5 pound that would have made it a weight-loss food. That was okay, not great, but she *loved* peanut butter. I believe in balance, so I said, "Look, Janet, we both know peanut butter is not optimal for your weight or your BBT, but it's a food that makes you really happy—and I want you to be happy! Feel free to have peanut butter once a week."

Now, we all have an inner three-year-old who hates to be told what to do, so of course Janet ignored me and had peanut butter two days later. This time, instead of losing 0.2 pound, she *gained* 0.2 pound, and her BBT dropped by 0.5 degree. She still couldn't believe that her beloved peanuts had this effect, so she ate peanut butter again the next day. This time she gained a pound and her BBT dropped a full point.

Janet got the picture. She went back to having peanut butter once a week, her weight loss resumed, and her thyroid remained in an optimal zone. She didn't have to give up one of her favorite foods—she just had to enjoy it in moderation. So please, trust me when I say that you will find many, many foods that you love and can rotate into your diet that will promote your best metabolic health! You just need to take it slow on the foods that are more challenging.

What's Going On with Your BBT?

Remember, your BBT will drop if you get too much exercise—that's one of the things we're trying to measure. However, other factors can also lower your BBT, so to get an accurate reading, make sure you take care of the following.

- **Get enough sleep**: If you need some sleep support, see page 62.
- **Keep stress in check**: Meditate, take SAM-e, or take some hops or lemon balm on a stressful day to mitigate the effects of cortisol. (See page 173.)
- **Avoid goitrogens**: Because these foods can lower your thyroid function, stick to the protocol on pages 192 and 193.
- **Women**: Note that your BBT will drop on the day your cycle starts and also after you ovulate. Tracking your cycle will help you plan your exercise. For example, if a half-hour run boosts your BBT and an hour run decreases it, schedule the half-hour run when your cycle starts. Using exercise to balance your BBT will help keep your metabolism humming for the most effective weight loss.

Your Daily To-Do List

- Eat until you're full at every meal.
- Even if you don't finish all the food, please make sure to have part of each recommended dish.
- Stay hydrated by drinking half your body weight in ounces. Drink between meals—45 minutes away from eating. Try to finish all of your water 45 minutes before dinner and do not have any water after dinner for best weight loss.
- Soup portions are 16 ounces for women, 20 ounces for men. Please do not have more.
  - **Women**: When seeds, nuts, or cheese is listed at any meal, please have 1 to 1.5 ounces. Animal protein portions are 4 to 6 ounces. Egg portion is 3 eggs.

- **Men**: When seeds, nuts, or cheese is listed at any meal, please have 2 to 3 ounces. Animal protein portions are 6 to 8 ounces. Egg portion is 4 eggs.
- Remember to dress your salad with lemon juice and EVOO, or with the vinaigrette of your choice (page 265).
- Approved fruits for breakfast cereal on The Metabolism Plan are blueberries, pears, and apples.
  - **Women**: Half a piece of fruit or ½ cup of blueberries.
  - **Men**: A whole piece of fruit or 1 cup of blueberries.

Your Morning Routine

- Take your BBT (see page 45 for instructions).
- Weigh yourself and record the results in your journal.
- After weighing, drink 16 ounces of fresh water with lemon juice.
- Take supplements as needed.

DAY 11: TEST INCREASED EXERCISE

This is an exciting day! You've been exercising for almost a week, and your body may be ready for a slightly bigger challenge. Or, if you're happy where you are, feel free to stay at your current level of duration and intensity—but then try some new types of exercise. One caveat, though. If you were reactive to your test food, stay with an approved exercise today. You can test increased exercise on your next test day.

Now, some of you have been wondering when you can take classes or work with your trainer again. Don't worry—this week is going to help get you there, because over the next 10 days, you can make your exercise either 20 percent *longer,* or 20 percent *more intensive.* We will be testing how your body reacts to even longer times—up to 90 minutes—during Days 21 to 30. If you pass those tests, it's back to class you go!

However, if you find by the end of this phase that your body does best with 20 minutes, at least for now, stick with a half-hour exercise class that has a nice cooldown at the end. Maybe you can work up to longer times later on.

Meanwhile, today, you have two options.

Option 1: Increase your exercise time by 20 percent.
OR
Option 2: Increase the amount of weight you lift by 20 percent.

I'm betting that you'll get an extra burst of endorphins and feel just terrific—but possibly, your body will say, politely but firmly, "No, thank you, I liked it better before." The scale and the thermometer will make your body's message clear. Since sleep, stress, or other factors could disrupt your results, we'll give you three chances. Increase your exercise by 20 percent on Days 11, 13, and 15. If your body says "No" all three days, then go back to what worked for you in the previous week.

BREAKFAST

Flax Granola (page 251) with approved fruit (see page 195)
Served with Silk Coconut Milk or Rice Dream
OR
Almond Grabbers (page 266) and approved fruit

LUNCH

Baby romaine with hard or soft goat cheese, carrots, and dried
    cranberries
Cream of Broccoli Soup (page 253)

SNACK

Trail Mix (page 267)
OR
Low-sodium potato chips
Women: 2 tablespoons almond butter
Men: 3 to 4 tablespoons almond butter

DINNER

Chicken with herbs of choice
Sautéed Zucchini Pasta (page 256) and Sunflower Pesto
    (page 262)
Baby romaine with radicchio and pomegranate

DAY 12: TEST A NEW VEGETABLE

Your low-reactive options are:

- potatoes
- Low-Reactive Tomato Sauce (page 261)
- snow peas
- Brussels sprouts.

I've given you these four options because they are very likely to work for you. Most people can manage them with no trouble, and if you can, too, you'll have another terrific option to rotate into the mix.

Generally, if your inflammation levels are high, your body may react poorly to many different foods. As you bring inflammation down, your digestion and immune system become stronger, enabling you to handle foods that triggered a reaction before. So whether or not you pass this test, don't worry. Many foods that don't work now almost certainly will work in the next 3 to 12 months, giving you a whole world of delicious foods to look forward to.

BREAKFAST

TMP Smoothie (page 248)
OR
Blueberry Compote (page 249)

LUNCH

Chicken Kale Soup (page 254)
Baby romaine with ¼ avocado and pumpkin seeds

SNACK

1 ounce Bare Apple Chips OR Apple Chips (page 269) with
optional Zucchini Noush (page 269)
OR
Trail Mix (page 267)

DINNER

Any protein you have tested and found friendly (for portion sizes,
see page 166)

Test a new vegetable—sautéed, steamed, or baked: ½ cup to
1 cup

Sautéed zucchini, yellow squash, and scallions

Baby romaine and pomegranate

DAY 13: TEST INCREASED EXERCISE WHILE ENJOYING
ANY FRIENDLY PROTEIN

Once again, you've got two options, depending on how your Day 11
went.

Option 1: If the Day 11 testing showed that your body liked
increased exercise, terrific! Pick another type of exercise that
works for you, and do it 20 percent longer or with 20 percent
more weight.

Option 2: If the Day 11 testing produced weight gain or lowered
your BBT, repeat the test. We want to be sure that the negative
result was because of the exercise and not due to sleep, stress,
or any other factor.

Meanwhile, for dinner, choose a protein that you've already tested
and found friendly.

BREAKFAST

Flax Granola (page 251) with a friendly fruit (see page 195)

Served with Silk Coconut Milk or Rice Dream

LUNCH

Leftover vegetables with sunflower seeds and ½ apple on a bed
of red leaf lettuce

Chicken Kale Soup (page 254)

SNACK

Trail Mix (page 267)
OR
Low-sodium potato chips

DINNER

Any protein that you have tested and found friendly
Baby romaine with grated beet and fresh dill
Sautéed kale and carrots

Wondering About Wheat?

So many of my clients stress about giving up wheat, pasta, and bread, so I'm going to tell you what I tell them: Don't worry! Bread is such a great comfort food, and I want you to be able to enjoy it. I promise, you will definitely be able to find some kind of bread or grain that works for you.

Wheat is what we first think of when we think of bread and pasta, and it's quite possible that you'll be able to make wheat a part of your diet. However, the following "alternative wheats" are often easier to digest.

- **Spelt** is a type of heirloom wheat. Like the more common form of wheat, it does contain gluten, but it's often much easier on your digestive tract. It has more protein than regular wheat, and more trace minerals, too.
- **Kamut** is another type of heirloom wheat that also contains gluten and is easier to digest than regular wheat. It likewise is better than regular wheat, both in protein content and in terms of trace minerals. Moreover, kamut is quite high in lipids (fats), which makes it taste rather buttery. Mmmm!
- **Einkorn** is the oldest type of wheat we know about—the only type that has never been hybridized. It does contain gluten, but in

a less dense form than regular wheat, and has less starch, which makes it easier on your gut.

You also might be able to digest regular wheat, especially after you have healed your gut and lowered your inflammation.

I personally like having my clients test spelt cereal first because it's like wheat, but so much easier to digest. If you pass spelt, there's a great chance you will be able to eat some sort of wheat. Another great way to test wheat is to order the crackers from Columbia County Bread and Flax (Resources); they are delicious, have no yeast, are sprouted, and are very low-gluten.

DAY 14: OPTIONAL TEST: BREAD OR SPELT

Aren't you excited? You get to test wheat today!

Of course, if you have celiac disease, or you know you've had a bad reaction to bread in the past, you can skip this test. You're the one who best knows your body and your history, so use your own judgment here.

But as you can see, The Metabolism Plan is *not* anti-gluten, as so many programs are. I think that some gluten in moderation can be perfectly fine for people without celiac disease, especially as you bring down your levels of inflammation and become healthier. Even if you choose not to test bread now, those among you without celiac disease might want to try it in three to six months.

BREAKFAST

Any breakfast you have tested and found friendly
OR
Women: 1 slice of bread with raw almond butter and ½ apple
Men: 2 slices of bread with raw almond butter and a whole
    apple
OR

Test Arrowhead Mills Spelt Cereal, adding 2 tablespoons of chia
seeds and sunflower seeds (for portion, see page 166)

LUNCH

Chicken Kale Soup (page 254)
Baby romaine with sunflower seeds and carrots

SNACK

1 ounce low-sodium potato chips
OR
Trail Mix (page 267)

DINNER

Approved protein
Zucchini Pasta (page 256) with scallions, basil, and grated
Manchego
Baby romaine with ¼ pear

DAY 15: TEST EXERCISE, EAT ANY FRIENDLY PROTEIN

Option 1: If your body is doing well with increased exercise,
terrific! Pick another type of exercise that works for you, or
repeat a favorite. Either way, exercise 20 percent longer or
with 20 percent more weight.

Option 2: If the Day 11 and Day 13 testing produced weight gain
or lowered your BBT, repeat the test. We want to be sure that
the negative result was because of the exercise and not due to
sleep, stress, or any other factor.

As on Day 13, you also want to choose a protein for dinner that
you already know is friendly. That way, you'll know for sure that your
results reflect your exercise test and not your reaction to a new type
of food. Remember to follow the guidelines for rotating proteins,
which you can find on page 175.

BREAKFAST

Blueberry Compote (page 249)
OR
TMP Smoothie (page 248)

LUNCH

Cream of Broccoli Soup (page 253)
Baby romaine with raw beet and pumpkin seeds

SNACK

Carrots with Vegan Creamy Kale Dip (page 270)
OR
Trail Mix (page 267)

DINNER

Chicken with Indian Spice Rub (page 258)
Sautéed kale with onions and yellow squash
Baby romaine and pomegranate

DAY 16: TEST CHICKPEAS *OR* TEST RICE AT LUNCH

It's time to jazz up those lunches a bit! If you do well with a cup of rice at lunch, that's great fuel on your workout days. Chickpeas open up a whole wide world as well, with tasty snacks like The Plan's Hummus (page 268)! Rice and chickpeas each yield approximately 5 grams of protein, but are a higher reactive test when combined.

Just to note, chickpeas tend to pair poorly with animal protein, and for some folks they cause gas when mixed with broccoli. Choose chickpeas that have 100 grams of sodium or less per serving. Goya and Whole Foods are both good options. Chickpeas do go wonderfully with kale, so that will be one of today's lunch options. Rice goes very well with seeds and vegetable proteins like broccoli and kale, so that will be your other lunchtime choice.

BREAKFAST

Flax Granola (page 251) with friendly fruit (see page 195)
Served with Silk Coconut Milk or Rice Dream

LUNCH

Chickpea option: Sautéed chickpeas with curry, carrots, and kale
Baby romaine with ¼ avocado and sunflower seeds
OR
Rice option: Sautéed kale with yellow squash served over 1 cup bas-
    mati rice and topped with pumpkin seed hummus (page 268)
Salad with grated beet and carrot

SNACK

Low-sodium potato chips
OR
½ apple and almond butter

DINNER

Any protein you have tested and found friendly
Steamed, roasted, or sautéed vegetables you have tested and
    found friendly
Baby romaine with radicchio

DAY 17: TEST EXERCISE

What you do on this day will depend on how your previous exercise
days have gone. I want you to have at least two forms of exercise
in your rotation, and, ideally, three. So bump up either the time or
intensity on an exercise you've already tested, or find a new exercise
to test. Remember, variety is the spice of life!

As always, eat a protein that you've already tested today, so that
you don't confuse your response to a new level of exercise with your
response to a new protein.

BREAKFAST

 Apple Streusel (page 249)
 OR
 Blueberry Compote (page 249)

LUNCH

 Chicken Kale Soup (page 254)
 Baby romaine with ¼ avocado, dried cranberries, and sunflower
  seeds

SNACK

 Spicy Roasted Pumpkin Seeds (page 267)
 OR
 Bare Apple Chips OR Apple Chips (page 269) and Zucchini
  Noush (page 269)

DINNER

 Friendly protein
 Vegetable Timbale (page 257)
 Baby romaine with grated beet and dill

DAY 18: TEST YOUR FAVORITE RESTAURANT

Tired of cooking? Well, today is your lucky day: You are going to start testing local restaurants so you can enjoy some nights out! Here are a few suggestions for how to make each restaurant experience positive and healthy.

 • **Order your friendly foods with no salt**. Here's my motto: If it's salty, send it back! If you can get the chef to leave out the salt, you can enjoy lots of foods from your favorite menus.
 • **Avoid the chicken**. I'm not saying there are no exceptions. But ordering chicken in a restaurant is usually a disaster. Know why? Sodium. Ugh. I can't tell you how many of my clients have suffered

through another boring "healthy" grilled chicken breast only to gain a pound. That's because chicken hides the taste of sodium very, *very* well. Also, chefs, bless their hearts, often try to make chicken tastier by using chicken stock to marinate the meat to give it more flavor. And guess what almost every commercially prepared chicken stock has? MSG, a.k.a. insta–weight gain.

• **Ask whether they use beef tenderizer.** Yes, it makes the meat more juicy. But guess what it contains? Yup, you guessed it, MSG. No go.

• **Go for the steak, grilled lamb, duck breast, or fish.** My clients usually do well with these foods, and if you've tested well for them at home, they'll probably work for you in a restaurant.

• **Choose the sashimi.** I find that sashimi is pretty golden, too—you just need to avoid the soy sauce. And yes, that means low-sodium soy sauce. When I eat sashimi, I just mix some water with my wasabi and go for the straight sinus clear! The pickled ginger is fine, too, but steer clear of the pink stuff, because there are major issues with the dye.

BREAKFAST

TMP Smoothie (page 248)
OR
Blueberry Compote (page 249)

LUNCH

Women: 1 cup roasted or steamed broccoli served on a bed of baby romaine with goat cheese and sunflower seeds
Men: 2 cups roasted or steamed broccoli served on a bed of baby romaine with carrots, goat cheese, and sunflower seeds
Women and Men: Lemon Basil Escarole Soup (page 254)

SNACK

1 ounce low-sodium potato chips with ⅛ cup homemade guacamole (page 270)

DINNER

Test a restaurant

OR

Choose any friendly dinner you have enjoyed.

DAY 19 AND DAY 20: TEST EXERCISE *OR* TEST COMBINATION EXERCISE

If any of your exercise test results have been unclear, today is a great day to repeat your test for more accurate data.

Want to bump it up a notch? Combine two approved exercises and work out for up to 45 minutes!

As for food, repeat your two favorite days thus far. It's a great time to use some leftovers, giving you time to prep for Days 21 to 30. (See the cooking hacks on page 212 for suggestions on how to get a lot of food ready for the coming phase.)

If You Want to Speed Up Your Weight Loss...

I'd like you to keep testing foods so that you can expand your choices and have more options for rotation. But if your top priority is losing weight as quickly as possible, test a new food only every fourth day. That gives you three days of guaranteed weight loss, plus a testing day where you might also lose weight.

Tips from the Experts—Jonathan Bailor, *New York Times*-bestselling author, Weight Loss Expert, and CEO of SANESolution.com

1. Exercise more muscle to get best results. To increase resistance and maximize the results of your workout without increasing the impact on your body, concentrate your effort on exercising all muscle fibers.

Why do people *ride* a bike to burn body fat instead of *drawing pictures* of bikes to burn body fat? After all, both activities exercise muscles!

We choose to ride a bike because doing so exercises more muscle (the large leg muscles) than drawing bikes (the small hand muscles). The more muscle we exercise, the better our results. Traditional exercise has gotten that much right.

However, we can do a lot better. Just as we get better results in less time by working more muscles within our body, we get even *better* results in even *less* time by exercising more of the individual fibers that make up our muscles.

2. Increase resistance to increase results. You can increase resistance by lifting heavier weights or otherwise pushing your body harder.

If we have more hair cut off when we get a haircut, we can get haircuts less often. That is not some too-good-to-be-true gimmick. That is common sense. The more hair that is cut off, the more time we need to grow it back.

Similarly, if we exercise more muscle, we can exercise less often, because more time is required to recover.

3. Engage in eccentric exercise.

Every resistance training exercise has two parts: increasing the resistance (for example, standing up) and decreasing the resistance (for example, sitting down). Increasing the resistance is called the *concentric* portion of the exercise—when the muscle contracts. Decreasing the resistance is called the *eccentric* portion of the exercise—when the muscle extends. *Lifting* weights—the concentric action—gets more attention in muscle magazines. But *lowering* weights—the eccentric action—gets more results in studies.

Enjoying Your New Metabolism

Now that you're two-thirds of the way through your Metabolism Plan, how are you feeling? I know *I* am excited for you, because you're finally getting the answers you've been looking for about what will and will not help you lose weight. You are doing an amazing job of figuring out how to be your best life coach!

We're almost there—but there is still one step to go. In the next section, "Fine-Tuning Your Plan," you are truly going to make this Metabolism Plan your own. You are going to figure out what to test, using the methods you now understand so well and taking complete charge of your own diet and exercise plan.

CHAPTER TEN

Days 21 to 30

Fine-Tuning Your Plan

This is the homestretch, and I am so proud of you! In this phase, you will increase your workouts by another 20 percent, up to a total of 90 minutes. That means you can test your favorite exercise classes or sessions with your trainer.

Have you found that some of your favorite exercises didn't pass? That's okay. Remember how, after two years of not running, I started sprinting again? Keep testing new types of exercise at the times and intensity you began with in Chapter 7 and gradually keep working your way up. Your goal is to find something fun (remember the kid on the playground!) that also makes your body happy. It's amazing how small tweaks, such as lowering or raising the amount of weight you lift by just 20 percent, can make a huge difference in how your body responds.

In this next phase, I am pushing you out of the nest so you can enjoy a bit of freedom. In other words, it's time to start making your own menus! After all, you'll be creating your own menus for the rest of your life. Let's get started now so you really get the feel of how to put together the foods your body loves.

The process is really quite simple. First, meet the protein requirements for each meal by choosing the proteins you like that work for you. Then plug in your friendly foods. And always remember that our motto is "rotate or react." In other words, don't repeat any food during the day, and don't eat any protein two days running. If you have kale and sunflower seeds at lunch on Monday, don't have kale and sunflower seeds at dinner or on Tuesday. Save them for Wednesday!

Does this sound like a lot to manage? Don't worry, I've made it super easy. This chapter will walk you through how to create a menu and give you some easy cooking hacks to keep you on track. You can also download my app "The Metabolism Planner" from my website, which will guide you through all 30 days (and beyond) and also help you program your menus.

Menu Creation Step by Step

- Create a list of all the foods that have worked for you.
- Eat one animal protein a day *at most*, unless you have successfully tested eating two animal proteins in one day. Remember to use the guide on page 175 to help you rotate your proteins.
- Eat one grain a day *at most*. In other words, you can have either rice or bread once a day. Try to rotate so that you have each type of carb every other day. You can test to see how you do with more carbs per day. If you pass it, I recommend saving your double carbs for workout days, when your extra exertion balances the increased consumption.
- Eat one bean serving a day *at most*.
- You can have multiple servings of seeds and nuts on any one day, but rotate the *types* of seeds and nuts as often as possible and never have the same type more than once a day. So if you have almonds for breakfast, have sunflower seeds for lunch; if you have chia seeds for breakfast, have pumpkin seeds for lunch.
- As you have been doing, women can have 1 to 1.5 ounces of cheese a day, while men can have 2 to 3 ounces of cheese a day.

Proteins

If you want to try more than one daily serving of animal protein, grains, beans, or cheese, use one of your test days to test two servings.

If you pass this test, have your double serving on the days you exercise, so that the extra activity balances the increased consumption.

Menu-Making for Women

Note: You can download this menu-making template and Days 1 to 30 from our website.

Protein Ranges

Breakfast: 10 to 40 grams of protein (use the higher end of the range if you are an athlete).

Lunch: 15 grams of protein (if you exercise for more than 90 minutes a day, boost protein at lunch to 25 grams).

Dinner: 25 to 60 grams of protein (most women do best with 35 to 40 grams).

Menu-Making for Men

Note: You can download this menu-making template and Days 1 to 30 from our website.

Protein Ranges

Breakfast: 15 to 60 grams of protein (use the higher end of the range if you are an athlete).

Lunch: 20 to 35 grams of protein (use the higher end of the range if you are an athlete).

Dinner: 40 to 70 grams of protein.

The Metabolism Plan Proteins

Broccoli: approximately 5 grams per cup of finely chopped cooked broccoli

Sunflower seeds: approximately 6 grams per ounce

Pumpkin seeds: approximately 9 grams per ounce

Almonds: approximately 7 grams per ounce

Cheese: approximately 6 to 8 grams per ounce (soft cheese will be less)

Chickpeas: approximately 6 grams per ½ cup

Rice: approximately 4 grams per 1 cup

Chia: approximately 5 grams per 2 tablespoons

Kale: 5 grams per 2 cups finely chopped cooked

Cream of Broccoli Soup: approximately 7 grams per 16 ounces

Chicken Kale Soup: approximately 10 grams per 16 ounces

Cooking Hacks for Days 21 to 30

- Pick a cooking day early in this phase and make Chicken Kale Soup (page 254), Cream of Broccoli Soup (page 253), and any other soup you love for easy meals. Remember, you can always make soup and freeze it in batches for days when you need something fast.

- Roast a chicken for the week.

- Chop all of your vegetables—broccoli, yellow squash, onions, zucchini, and kale—and store them. Or buy prechopped vegetables, which you can do in many stores. As we've seen, even if you lose a little nutritional value, the stress relief you gain more than makes up for it! Frozen vegetables are also an easy and often inexpensive way to get those dinner veggies ready. Frozen vegetables are picked when they are ripe, so can often be a better choice than vegetables that are grown thousands of miles away and picked before they ripen. Remember, the more time a vegetable has to grow in the sun and in dirt, the more nutrients you get!

- Make a batch or two of zucchini pasta and keep it handy in the fridge for the week.

- Prepare some sauces from the Recipes section on pages 258 to 264 and keep them on hand, so you can add them to your roast chicken or vegetables for extra convenience.

- Many grocery stores have salad bars where you can pick up roasted, grilled, or steamed vegetables. Do some hunting around in your local area—you can certainly get them at Whole Foods. Most groceries have roast chicken as well. This is the a perfect time to start testing more convenient methods of cooking so you can bust loose out of the kitchen if you'd like to! Let's say you know that every time you eat chicken at home, you lose half a pound. So if you test a rotisserie chicken from a local store, you should lose half a pound, too. If you don't, then guess what? Too much sodium! That's okay, you can keep looking until you find the grocery store selling chicken that you *can* eat. Many grocery stores now label their rotisserie chicken as being salt-free, so try those places first.

- Happy to stay at home and cook? Return to some of the recipes from this book or try some new ones from *The Plan Cookbook* and invite friends and family over for dinner. It will never feel like a diet if you are sharing delicious food with people you love.

Fruit

Choose the fruits you have already been eating—apples, blueberries, dried cranberries, pears, and pomegranates. Your smoothie, compote, and streusel each count as one serving.

Women: Up to 1.5 servings of fruit per day

Men: Up to 2 servings of fruit per day

Seeds

Chia seeds and flaxseeds are great proteins full of many nutrients, which makes them a great addition to your diet. However, they also have a tendency to expand, so I find that they do best on an empty stomach—that is, at breakfast, when you haven't eaten anything for several hours.

Does that mean you can't have a chia-rich lunch? No, just know that it is a mild test. This is an easy one: If you feel bloated after a lunch with chia, it didn't work for you.

Portions

All the portions in the meal plans and recipes are the least reactive amounts. If you would like to use larger portions, please test them so you know whether they produce weight gain, weight stabilization, or symptoms.

Natural Sugars

I want you to eat the foods you love—and that includes sweet foods. But I don't want you to overdo it. Remember, when you eat any food—even a friendly one that has passed a test—moderation is the key.

I've found that most people do well with limiting their intake of natural sugars, such as fruit and winter squashes. Roasted vegetables fall into this category as well, since a vegetable's natural sugars are increased when the vegetable is cooked for a long time. Find your own balance: Begin by limiting roasted veggies and winter squash to a total of twice a week—that is, two portions of one, or one portion of both. You can expand as you find out what works for your body. As you test your own choices, you'll fine-tune your own personal Metabolism Plan. Remember, when you start exercising for more than 75 minutes, your body may love more natural sugars, carbs, or protein.

Combination Tests

Combining animal protein plus either grain or legumes at the same meal is something you have to test. For example, you might want to test chicken (animal protein) plus chickpeas (legume) or rice (grain). Or perhaps you'd like to test a combination of eggs (animal protein) plus bread (grain). Combining coconut milk and animal proteins is also something you need to test. Interestingly, fish and seafood tend to combine less reactively with both coconut milk and rice.

Digestion

In winter we always have either a cooked vegetable or a soup with lunch to aid digestion. Cooked foods are easier to digest than raw ones because fiber gives your digestive track more of a workout, and the cooking process reduces that fiber. Soups are easier to absorb and digest than cooked foods because they contain even less fiber, but don't have soup at dinner. Too much fluid at the end of the day hampers digestion.

Dinner always includes cooked vegetables and a raw vegetable salad, because raw vegetables contain enzymes that aid digestion. You want to keep an eye on having only raw vegetables at a meal, however, since their higher fiber content makes them harder to digest. (Your digestive tract likes the enzymes and likes the fiber in raw vegetables—but *too much* fiber can become a bit too much of a challenge.) Remember, anytime you hamper digestion, you slow weight loss. Always support your best digestion, and you are rewarded with optimal mood, body, and health.

When summer rolls around—think the heat of July and August— you may be able to digest raw salads beautifully. Remember how I told you that traditional Chinese medicine considers some lettuces to be "cold vegetables"? Your body can tolerate "cold vegetables" better in the heat of summer, so try a raw salad and see how you feel. If you bloat, that's a sign to add in more cooked vegetables.

And don't think, just because you live in a temperate climate, that you don't have a "cold season"—it's all relative! When I lived in balmy Hawaii, 70 degrees felt freezing to me! Some of my Wisconsin friends take off their winter jackets when the temperature reaches the high 40s. Either way, you want cold vegetables in *your* warm season, and hot soups with cooked veggies in *your* cold season. Your digestion will be happier, and so will you.

Retesting Foods

How do you know when to retest a food? It's all based on your handy scale! Let's say you gain half a pound after testing peanut butter. Based on your weight gain, you haven't had a terrible reaction—the food triggers some inflammation, but not an overwhelming amount. In that case, retest in three to six months. You were probably just overdoing the PB&Js. Now, let's say you test fish and you gain 2 pounds. Weight gain of that magnitude is a loud and clear sign from your body that you should take a *long* break from that food. Wait a year and then retest. And even if you pass, limit its use to once a week!

Bored with Your Repertoire?

Here are some testing options to liven it up:

- Test a new vegetable or fruit.
- Test a new vegetable protein or something to beef up protein in your smoothies.
- Test larger portions of proteins to fuel your workouts. This will be helpful as you increase your exercise times and intensify your weight training.
- Test two servings of carbs or larger portions to fit your increased cardio/workout needs.
- Try some of our sauces from pages 258 to 264 to add zing to your dishes.

Adding Carbs

One of our mantras on The Metabolism Plan is that when you find a new friendly carb, plug it in on your workout days, especially now that you are increasing intensity. Research has shown that eating slow-digesting carbs such as whole grains at breakfast and lunch leads to lower insulin levels and more fat burned during the day. So if you haven't tested any grains yet, please do!

Adding Animal Protein to Your Lunches

What about animal protein at lunch? Your chicken soup passes, of course, but generally, animal proteins at lunch are hard to digest. Feel free to test it, though, and see how you feel.

Build Your Own Menu

Here's a blueprint to help you build your own Metabolism Plan menus with a list of your low-reactive protein choices. On exercise days, use only foods you have already tested.

BREAKFAST

Easy sources of protein are flax, seeds, nuts and nut butters, and cereals. Limit flax to two times a week now.

Optional: Add fruit

Women: 10 to 40 grams of protein (Stay at the lower end of this spectrum unless you are an athlete.)

Men: 15 to 60 grams of protein

LUNCH

Soup and salad with vegetarian proteins is ideal. Build a salad from friendly vegetables, seeds, nuts, and perhaps some cheese.

When the weather is below 75 degrees, always add a soup or cooked vegetable to enhance digestion.

Women: Aim for a total of 15 to 25 grams of protein taken from the low-reactive protein chart on page 14. (Remain at the lower end of the spectrum unless you are an athlete.)

Men: Aim for a total of 20 to 35 grams of protein taken from the low-reactive protein chart on page 14. (Remain at the lower end of the spectrum unless you are an athlete.)

SNACK

Your favorite friendly snack

DINNER

Friendly protein

Friendly salad

Friendly cooked vegetable

In winter, always include cooked vegetables plus a raw vegetable salad, since raw vegetables contain enzymes that support digestion. You want to support your digestion at night so you can go on to get a good sleep.

Women: 25 to 60 grams of protein
Men: 40 to 70 grams of protein

Your Daily To-Do List

- Eat until you're full at every meal.
- Even if you don't finish all the food, please make sure to have part of each recommended dish.
- Stay hydrated by drinking half your body weight in ounces. Drink between meals—45 minutes away from eating. Try to finish all of your water 45 minutes before dinner and do not have any water after dinner for best weight loss.

Your Morning Routine

- Take your BBT (see page 45 for instructions).
- Weigh yourself and record the results in your journal.
- After weighing, drink 16 ounces of fresh water with lemon juice.
- Take supplements as needed.

DAY 21: TEST INCREASED EXERCISE

How exciting! Your first day to make your own menu. This is your chance to put foods together in your very own way, while also testing increased exercise. If you are happy where you are with your exercise levels, then stay at that level and use this day to test foods or some element of your lifestyle, such as how much sleep you get. Or just coast and relax!

If you decide to test increased intensity and your body likes it, you can go on to increase a different type of exercise on Day 23. However, if you increase exercise today, and your weight and BBT respond poorly, you have two more days—Days 23 and 25—to repeat the test, just to make completely sure that stress, sleep, or some other factor didn't interfere with your results.

For exercise, you have three options:

- Stay with your current level.
- Increase your amount of exercise time or intensity by 20 percent.
- Increase the amount of weight you lift by 20 percent.

If you decide to increase exercise, make sure to test only exercises that you have passed already. So if you have been doing 20 minutes of kettlebells, you can now increase to 25 minutes of kettlebells. (Yes, I know, technically, a 20 percent increase would be 24 minutes, but please—round up!) Or you can add 20 percent more weight—so you could bump those 8-pound weights to a rounded-up 10 pounds.

As far as hydration goes, drink during exercise until you quench your thirst; then drink your regular hydration amount throughout the rest of the day. The rough rule of thumb is to drink an extra 8 ounces of water for every 30 minutes of exercise.

I also want you to stretch. I have some great videos on my website that you can choose to incorporate after your workouts or the next day. And for my exercise nuts, don't worry—gentle stretching (and meditation, too!) will not count toward your exercise time and can actually help to lower cortisol.

BREAKFAST

Easy sources of protein are flax, seeds, nuts and nut butters, and cereals.

Optional: Add fruit

LUNCH

Soup and salad with your approved proteins

When the weather is below 75 degrees, always add a soup or cooked vegetable to enhance digestion.

SNACK

Your favorite snack

DINNER

Friendly protein
Friendly salad
Friendly cooked vegetable

Running Longer—and Smarter

Now you can run longer if you'd like—yay! That means you need to start prepping your body so you don't get injured. You want to do only quick stretches of 10 seconds or less before your run and save the long stretches for later.

Unless you're training for a marathon, you may want to skip super-long runs. Sprinting will build more type II muscle fibers so that you burn more calories later. The upside? You'll become faster, too!

DAY 22: TEST A NEW VEGETABLE

Remember, if you want to concentrate on weight loss and you have enough friendly foods in your roster for now, you can skip this test day and test something new later. If you do want to avoid testing for now, try different sauces or herbs to add some excitement to your diet and your taste buds. Remember that herbs have powerful flavor and healing benefits, so something as simple as adding rosemary to your lamb or dill on your salad can go a long way!

If you do want to test a vegetable, your low-reactive options are:

- potatoes
- Low-Reactive Tomato Sauce (page 261)
- snow peas

- Brussels sprouts
- cooked fennel.

Of course, you can choose another vegetable—just be aware that these five are the most likely to pass! If you already passed snow peas on your vegetable test, there's a better chance that you will pass snap peas or green beans, so you might move on to them. If you choose to test a goitrogen from the list on pages 191–192 and you pass it, please limit it to once a week.

BREAKFAST

Easy sources of protein are flax, seeds, nuts and nut butters, and cereals.
Optional: Add fruit

LUNCH

Soup and salad with your approved vegetarian proteins: vegetables, nuts, seeds, and cheese. When the weather is below 75 degrees, always add a soup or cooked vegetable to enhance digestion.

SNACK

Your favorite friendly snack

DINNER

Friendly protein
Friendly salad
Friendly cooked vegetable

DAY 23: DAY OFF *OR* TEST EXERCISE

Okay, you might have gotten the idea by now that I think we are all working a little too hard, so I'm pushing for you to take a day off. Yes! A day off! Your body needs time to rest, reset, and get used to your new way of eating. With no new foods to test and a day off from exercise, your body can focus on bringing down the inflammation and repairing inflamed tissues.

I'd love you to make this a "me day" in some way. Do you have a chance to get a massage, take a walk somewhere lovely, or relax with a good book and a glass of wine? Is there someone you've been wanting to talk to for a while—a friend, a relative, someone you just don't get to hang out with very often?

Even if you're rocking your usual busy schedule with work, home, and family, take a few moments to breathe deep and appreciate your renewed health. As we learned in Chapter 3, stress has a biochemical effect on your metabolism and your weight. We're not stressing your body with new foods or exercise today, so any more de-stressing is all the better!

Don't want to take a day off? That's okay, too! You have four options:

- Retest the exercise from Day 21 if you didn't pass it.
- Stay with your current level of exercise, or stay with week 1 or 2.
- Increase the amount of exercise time or intensity by 20 percent.
- Increase the amount of weight you lift by 20 percent.

BREAKFAST

Easy sources of protein are flax, seeds, nuts and nut butters, and cereals.

Optional: Add fruit

LUNCH

Soup and salad with your approved vegetarian proteins: vegetables, nuts, seeds, and cheese. When the weather is below 75 degrees, add a soup or cooked vegetable to enhance digestion.

SNACK

Your favorite friendly snack

DINNER

Friendly protein
Friendly salad
Friendly cooked vegetable

Wielding the Weight

Training with heavy weights for 4 to 6 reps definitely builds strength. But remember, you can't keep pushing harder and heavier. It's all about a concept known as *periodization*. You should aim for periods of heavy weight training alternating with periods of lighter weights and more reps. Scientists at Baylor University have found that too much training with heavy weights too often can actually inhibit muscle growth.

DAY 24: OPTIONAL: TEST A NEW VEGETARIAN PROTEIN

Great choices to test are hemp hearts, chickpeas, lentils, and fresh mozzarella (hello, one step closer to pizza!). This will add some welcome diversity to your lunches and snacks! Or, if you'd prefer to focus on weight loss, just stick with foods you know are friendly so you can be sure to lose some more weight.

BREAKFAST

Easy sources of protein are flax, seeds, nuts and nut butters, and cereals.
Optional: Add fruit

LUNCH

Soup and salad with your approved vegetarian proteins: vegetables, nuts, seeds, and cheese. When the weather is below 75 degrees, always add a soup or cooked vegetable to enhance digestion.

SNACK

Your favorite friendly snack

DINNER

Friendly protein
Friendly salad
Friendly cooked vegetable

DAY 25: INCREASE EXERCISE BY 20 PERCENT, *OR* TEST EXERCISING IN THE EARLY MORNING OR EVENING

Okay, folks, for those of you who have been wanting to get back to that 5:30 a.m. boot camp or to work out *after* work instead of before, now's your chance! Try the alternate time and see how your body likes it. If you're exercising after 5 p.m., make sure to spend time in deep long stretches after exercise, better yet with deep breathing, to decrease stress and rebalance cortisol levels.

However, if you haven't yet increased your exercise, make sure you test *either* extra exercise—up to 90 minutes—*or* a new time, so that you know exactly what your body is responding to. Test those things separately, so you get good, solid results.

Of course, if you failed the test on Day 21 and this is your third day of testing, stick with your retest. You can always test increased exercise or alternate times later.

Other exercise options:

- Stay with your current level or decrease back to week 1 or week 2.
- Increase the amount of exercise time or intensity by 20 percent.
- Increase the amount of weight you lift by 20 percent.

BREAKFAST

Easy sources of protein are flax, seeds, nuts and nut butters, and cereals.
Optional: Add fruit

LUNCH

Soup and salad with your approved vegetarian proteins: vegetables, nuts, seeds, and cheese. When the weather is below
75 degrees, always add a soup or cooked vegetable to
enhance digestion.

SNACK

Your favorite friendly snack

DINNER

Friendly protein
Friendly salad
Friendly cooked vegetable

Biking Benefits and Tips

Did you know that by shifting your position in the saddle of a bicycle,
you can emphasize different muscle groups? Moving forward targets
your quads, while moving back emphasizes your hamstrings and glutes.

If you're gearing up for a longer trip like a century ride (100 miles
or more), here's the best way to build muscle, speed, and stamina.
Add 10 miles to each ride until you hit the higher numbers, like 80,
and see how you do. This will allow you keep tweaking your hydration and dietary needs to fit your new level of activity.

DAY 26: TEST A NEW RESTAURANT

That's right, I am shoving you out in the cold again. Now, of course
you don't *have* to go eat out. You can order in—did you try that
sashimi yet? Or, of course, you can cook at home. But I do want you
to start finding a way to make The Metabolism Plan a way of life, and
there's *nothing* better than going out, finding a restaurant you love,
and continuing to lose weight by eating there. An empty sink free of

dishes is also pretty awesome! There are at least five restaurants in a two-mile radius that I know work for me. I want you to have that experience, too. So reward yourself for all your hard work and get out of the kitchen!

Of course, your prep and the restaurant's prep can be worlds apart, especially because restaurants tend to use way too much salt. So some foods that tested fine at home might not work when you eat out. (Especially chicken! See page 204.) Still, many restaurants *will* work with you, and when you know which they are, you can rotate eating at home and eating out while continuing to lose weight. Bonus!

So what should your protocol be for restaurant testing? First, make sure you ask for your meal to be prepared without salt. Next, I want you to eat a full meal, but not to test any new foods. Save that for home! However, if you now know that you do well with, say, wheat, mozzarella, and tomato sauce, it's time to test your favorite thin-crust pizza at a great Italian restaurant. Have it with a salad, maybe some sautéed broccoli, a nice red, and call it a happy night.

Then, of course, if you lose weight, this meal at this restaurant is friendly. If you gain weight, don't let that stop you from eating out! Just try a new restaurant next time.

BREAKFAST

Easy sources of protein are flax, seeds, nuts and nut butters, and cereals.

Optional: Add fruit

LUNCH

Soup and salad with your approved vegetarian proteins: vegetables, nuts, seeds, and cheese. When the weather is below 75 degrees, always add a soup or cooked vegetable to enhance digestion.

SNACK

Your favorite friendly snack

DINNER

Friendly protein
Friendly salad
Friendly cooked vegetable

DAY 27: TEST EXERCISE INCREASED BY 20 PERCENT AND FOR UP TO 90 MINUTES

If you want to be doing a longer or more intense workout, this is your day to find out whether your thyroid likes the idea as much as you do! If you like, you can increase your exercise intensity by 20 percent, and feel free to exercise for up to 90 minutes. If you don't pass this test after three tries, you can always retest in three months. If your BBT and weight respond really badly, however, you might focus, at least for now, on finding other activities. Who knows? You might fall in love with a whole different approach to working out.

Of course, if you don't want to increase your exercise at this time, you don't have to. Here are your options for today:

- Stay with your current level or decrease back to week 1 or week 2.
- Increase the amount of exercise time or intensity by 20 percent.
- Increase the amount of weight you lift by 20 percent.

BREAKFAST

Easy sources of protein are flax, seeds, nuts and nut butters, and cereals.
Optional: Add fruit

LUNCH

Soup and salad with your approved vegetarian proteins: vegetables, nuts, seeds, and cheese. When the weather is below 75 degrees, always add a soup or cooked vegetable to enhance digestion.

SNACK

Your favorite friendly snack

DINNER

Friendly protein
Friendly salad
Friendly cooked vegetable

Learning a New Sport or Skill

If you're not loving your workout—or if you've been doing it forever—I want you to start exploring and find something you love to do that is new and challenging for your body. I get it—sometimes learning something new can be hard. But trust me, you want to get over that fear of showing up at a class where you don't know the moves or starting your ski skills on the bunny slope, because learning a new athletic skill can be empowering in so many ways, and you don't want to deprive yourself of the opportunity.

I remember how hard it was for my stepdaughter, Ella, to learn how to ride a bike. Once she figured it out, though, her confidence increased—and suddenly, she was having fun and feeling like queen of the neighborhood! I want you to have the same kind of fun.

Mastering new skills does so much for our spirit and for our entire body as well, from our brain to our muscles to our neurological system. Learning a new exercise actually stimulates cognitive function and helps prevent memory loss. So don't concentrate on how you're not doing it 100 percent, but rather on the fact that you *are* doing it. Bravo for you!

DAY 28: NO TEST

Instead of a test day I want you to create a friendly day, and I'll tell you why. I want you to have at least 20 solid days that you can always come back to when you need to lower inflammation. Too many people rely on the cleanse to quickly recalibrate after a reactive day or weekend. Yes, that's an option, but I want you to know that any day you want, you can lose weight and heal by just eating normally. So please compile all of your favorite friendly foods so far and make this a day where you lose weight like a rock star and eat all of your favorite foods. I call this my "French fry and cheese day."

BREAKFAST

Easy sources of protein are flax, seeds, nuts and nut butters, and cereals.
Optional: Add fruit

LUNCH

Soup and salad with your approved vegetarian proteins: vegetables, nuts, seeds, and cheese. When the weather is below 75 degrees, add a soup or cooked vegetable to enhance digestion.

SNACK

Your favorite friendly snack

DINNER

Friendly protein
Friendly salad
Friendly cooked vegetable

DAY 29: OPTIONAL: TEST BACK-TO-BACK EXERCISE, PART 1

All you exercise lovers have been waiting for this day! Over Days 29 and 30, you can test how your body responds to exercising two days in a row. Aren't you excited to see what this test is going to reveal?

So what happens if it doesn't work out? Does that mean you can *never* work out two days in a row? The answer is that you can most certainly work out two days in a row; you just might not want to do it every week. Just like you, I am balancing my life, my work, and my fitness goals. And sometimes that means that I have to work out on both Saturday and Sunday. That also means that when my stress levels are high, I am consistently up 0.6 pound on Monday. When stress levels are low, I can exercise on Saturdays and Sundays with no inflammatory response. But I *always* know why, and that's what's important. If that happens to you, too, I want you to understand why that number appears on your scale and what you can do about it. So, on the hectic weeks where work is crazy, I know I should take Sunday off and let the inflammation subside. Do I always do it? Not always, but I always know what to do and I also know that it's only when you have inflammatory day after inflammatory day that you start to set yourself up for trouble. So find the balance that works for you.

Of course, you don't *have* to test back-to-back exercise! As always, I want you to pick the approach that is right for *you*. Your options today:

- Stay with your current level or decrease back to week 1 or week 2.
- Increase the amount of exercise time or intensity by 20 percent.
- Increase the amount of weight you lift by 20 percent.

BREAKFAST

Easy sources of protein are flax, seeds, nuts and nut butters, and cereals.

Optional: Add fruit

LUNCH

Soup and salad with your approved vegetarian proteins: vegetables, nuts, seeds, and cheese. When the weather is below 75 degrees, always add a soup or cooked vegetable to enhance digestion.

SNACK

Your favorite friendly snack

DINNER

Friendly protein
Friendly salad
Friendly cooked vegetable

DAY 30: OPTIONAL: TEST BACK-TO-BACK EXERCISE, PART 2

If you decide to do exercise two days in a row, you might get the best results if you do a different type of exercise on the second day. For example, many of my clients do really well having a yoga day after weight training or running. If you're training your upper body one day, maybe do lower body or plyometrics the next day.

Try to think of your body holistically. To me that means considering how your body responds and creating a well-rounded regimen that supports total health. Rotating exercise will also help to keep you injury-free, which keeps you in the game longer. Last but not least, a well-rounded program will give you better body composition!

If you don't choose to do back-to-back exercise today, why not test another food? You might enjoy adding one more choice to your roster. If you're feeling adventurous, check out *The Plan Cookbook* and find a dish you'd love to make. Test one of the ingredients in that dish if it's not already on your friendly list.

BREAKFAST

Easy sources of protein are flax, seeds, nuts and nut butters, and cereals.
Optional: Add fruit

LUNCH

Soup and salad with your approved vegetarian proteins: vegetables, nuts, seeds, and cheese. When the weather is below 75 degrees, always add a soup or cooked vegetable to enhance digestion.

SNACK

Your favorite friendly snack

DINNER

Friendly protein
Friendly salad
Friendly cooked vegetable

Tips from The Experts: Dr. Steven Zodkoy, Author of *Misdiagnosed: The Adrenal Fatigue Link*

If you have been suffering from heightened levels of cortisol for an extended period of time, you may have adrenal fatigue. Adrenal fatigue changes the natural biochemistry of the body. The main changes are a heightened base cortisol level, increased glucose, and a minimized cortisol response to extra stress (exercise). These changes make the sufferer more prone to anxiety and weight gain.

The key to exercising with adrenal fatigue is a mild exercise routine, which can include walking, swimming, or biking—all are low impact to minimize inflammation. A good rule of thumb is to keep the heart rate between 75 and 85 beats per minute and to limit exercise to 20 minutes max until adrenal health is restored.

Tips from The Experts: Andia Winslow, Professional Athlete and Master Certified Fitness Professional

Tips for Runners

Interval training helps to improve overall cardiovascular fitness, speed, and race endurance. Here are some suggestions for improving your form, which will help you get better results—better times, stronger muscles, fewer injuries—and also help you enjoy the whole process more.

- Keep your eyes on the horizon, looking in the direction of your intended run. Your eyeline dictates your body line and the direction of your energy.
- Keep your jaw and face relaxed. Any tension in your jaw will permeate to your neck, shoulders, and arms, and eventually throughout your entire body, causing a restricted stride.
- Maintain a neutral neck. Imagine a tennis ball or fist space between your chin and chest. This also helps to relieve tension.
- Maintain supple shoulders that are down away from your ears.
- Keep your arms moving forward and back, not round and round across your body. What your arms do, your legs do. Any potential twisting in the upper body will translate into inefficient twisting in the lower body. Save the salsa dancing for the club on Friday night!

Reaching the Finish Line

Wow. You've done it! You have completely transformed your life. You've lost weight, boosted your energy, and rid yourself of symptoms that plagued you for years. You've improved your health, digestion, hormones, and immune system. You've learned how to get the sleep you need and how to manage stress. You've put yourself on the road to health, now and for the rest of your life.

You've also strengthened and balanced your metabolism, which is the best possible news, because now you will be able to lose weight until you reach your target. Then you can continue to maintain that healthy weight, now and for the rest of your life. What could be better?

So many people tell me that going through The Metabolism Plan is like being in one of those snow globes where their world is turned completely upside down and shaken up. Now the snow has settled and you are steady on your feet. Now you understand why you were having so many rough days before, days when you thought you were eating so healthy and doing the right thing, and yet your body seemed to betray you. Now you understand that those "betrayals" were actually your body's way of saying "I love you."

In the next chapter, you'll find out what you need to stay on this path, so that you can reach your optimal weight if you haven't already and attain your optimal health for life. But first, take a proud and joyful moment to pat yourself on the back. You've found the answers to the questions you had about what makes you gain weight or feel sick, and you've learned how to hear and understand when your body talks to you. And you know that from here on in, you will always have the power to take charge of your health, your weight, and your metabolism.

You're now in the driver's seat—time to make magic!

Part Three

YOUR METABOLISM PLAN FOR LIFE

CHAPTER ELEVEN

Your Dream Body

You did it, and you are really on your way! You've completed the 30 days of your Metabolism Plan, and now you have a really clear idea of what types of foods and exercise are perfect for your body. Better yet, you know how to test any type of food or exercise to find out for sure what works best *for you.*

This is huge, my dear friends. You are now in control of your weight, and you know exactly how to take charge of your health. The knowledge you have acquired will support you for the rest of your life.

Now, that doesn't mean the diet and exercise that work today will work forever. After all, your body keeps changing. Maybe today your body likes beef. In a year, your body might tell you, "Enough of beef—I'm ready for some fish!" The following year, you might find you need lamb. It's a never-ending process of growth and change.

Likewise, today your body might love Pilates. In one year, it might be ready to switch to weight training. The important thing is to keep listening to your body and letting it guide you.

So here's the best news of all: *You are now 100 percent able to do this!* How do I know? Because while your body's needs may change over time, the testing methodology of The Metabolism Plan doesn't.

With this knowledge, you will continue to lose weight until you reach your ideal healthy weight, and then you will be able to easily maintain that weight. For life. I promise.

Now, I often have people ask me, "Do I have to use the scale and take my BBT daily?" The answer is, it's up to you. I don't expect most people to keep taking their BBT daily after the 30 days unless they are trying to work on thyroid and endocrine issues that are still unresolved. So maybe just break out the thermometer when you are trying a new sport or doing endurance work, like training for a marathon. You can do the same thing with the scale once you stop testing foods. If you start to notice that your clothes aren't fitting the way they used to, bring out the scale and start retesting. Or you can just weigh yourself daily as I do. I'm always so intrigued by what my body is telling me daily, and the scale helps me listen. You can choose your own ways of listening, with or without the scale.

To get you ready for full independence, in this chapter I will:

- give you some overall guidelines for creating friendly menus by showing you how to rotate your foods throughout the week.
- tell you what to do if you hit a plateau.
- show you how to respond if you suddenly start gaining weight.

I also want to assure you that if you need any additional help—for any aspect of The Metabolism Plan whatsoever—my wonderful staff and I are always at your service. The Metabolism Plan team is a warm community, and we are always here for you.

Meanwhile, let's go over the last few things you need to know for now, next year, and the rest of your life.

Rotation Rules

You've tested quite a few foods in your 30 days, but I know you have lots more you want to test. That's terrific! You've got two options.

Option 1: To expand your food choices, test foods every other
   day.
Option 2: To speed up weight loss, test foods every fourth day.

The choice is yours. Testing foods more often means that you will
build up a list of friendly foods faster—foods that you know will help
you lose weight and maintain a healthy weight.

Testing foods less often means that for at least three days out of
four, you will continue to lose weight. This tends to work better if
you have 30 pounds or more to lose. Even so, please keep testing,
because you need a wide variety of foods to choose from for your
best health and weight. I don't want you sticking to just a few foods
for the next several months, let alone the rest of your life. You'll get
bored, you'll feel restricted, and you'll deprive your body of a world
of nutrients that might be exactly what you need for optimal health.

By now you are quite familiar with our slogan, "rotate or react"!
You can't follow it, though, unless you have enough foods in your
arsenal so that every day you can have 5 to 7 items that you did not
eat the day before. Even a friendly food that you've been eating for
months with no problem can turn unfriendly if you eat it too often,
especially if you eat it two or three days in a row. So let's set some
goals to keep you from turning your friendly foods into your enemies:

- **Use the animal protein rotation chart on page 175**. Your golden
  rule: Don't repeat animal proteins two days in a row. Animal proteins are the foods most likely to set off an inflammatory reaction,
  so we want to be extra careful not to overdo any one of them.
  Using the rotation chart will keep those friendly proteins friendly!
- **Eat any particular friendly grain no more than every other day**.
  Next to animal proteins, grains have the highest chance to be
  reactive. So don't overdo them, either. If you enjoy a stir-fry
  with rice on Monday, don't have rice again until Wednesday.
  If you can eat bread, then have it on Tuesday, Thursday, and

Saturday. I personally find it easiest to just tag each day of the week with the foods I can have that day—"rice on Monday, Wednesday and Friday; bread on Tuesday, Thursday, and Saturday." That way I have less thinking and less planning, and my mind is free for more important things—like choosing the right wine!

- **Try to never have any vegetable more than three days in a row.** Vegetables are probably the least reactive type of food, but I still don't want you to repeat them too often. Luckily, I've got an easy suggestion for you: Make a big batch of sautéed vegetables with no sauce. On the first day, heat it up with a sauté of ginger and garlic. On the second, heat it up and add the Spicy Almond Satay (page 259). On the third, warm it up and add dill and lemon. Now you've also cut down on cooking, which is a major bonus! Then make a new batch of completely different vegetables for your next three days and continue to rotate the sauces.
- **Every week, aim for one seed-free day, one dairy-free day, and perhaps one meat-free day.** Think Meatless Monday, for example.

These rotation rules may seem complicated now when you're reading this, but when you do The Plan and see what feels best for you, this is going to be second nature, I promise. It's not like these are rules you can *never* break. But the more you follow them, the more you are setting yourself up for success.

Why is rotation so important?

Well, it just so happens that every food contains dozens—maybe even hundreds—of biochemical compounds. The odds are that your body is not going to react well with *some* of the compounds present in every single food. In other words, even the friendliest of foods have some unfriendly components. These unfriendly components— even in tiny amounts—can be challenging to your body, especially if, like most of us, you are already leading a busy, stressful life and, like all of us, you are living in a world overloaded with industrial chemicals that requires your body to carry a growing toxic burden.

So our goal is to minimize the number of times your body has to metabolize *any* unfriendly compound. That way, your body can do a better job of digesting and absorbing everything you eat, and you are less likely to develop a food sensitivity.

Here's your golden rule: Friendly foods will work for you—but they can become inflammatory if you eat them too often. So follow the rotation guidelines on pages 239 and 240, on page 175 (for animal proteins) and on pages 191 and 192 (for goitrogens).

Or, if you prefer your golden rules short and sweet:

Rotate or react. (You were expecting that one, weren't you?)

Keep Retesting Every Six Months

Okay, so you've got your rotations all set up. You know which foods are friendly and which cause you to gain weight, develop symptoms, and otherwise feel lousy. You know which foods you can eat once a week and which foods you can enjoy more often. You've got your weekly routine down pat, and it's really working for you. You're all set, right?

Well, yes. And no. You can forget about testing foods for a while. But I do want you to retest your friendly foods every 6 to 12 months.

Why? Because, your body keeps changing, which means your foods need to keep changing, too. After all, your body is a dynamic biochemical system that responds with intricate precision to every bite of food, every minute of exercise, every moment of stress. As a complex living organism, you are growing and changing every single day, and that means that your food requirements evolve also.

Some of this is precisely because you are making up for years of being out of balance. Maybe when you started your Metabolism Plan, you were deficient in selenium and iodine, so scallops and cod were your friendly foods. Then, in maybe a year, your selenium and iodine are back in balance, but you need more iron. Suddenly scallops and cod become unfriendly, while steak and lamb are exactly what your body wants.

Or suppose you've just been through a significant crisis. Maybe someone you loved was ill, or you had to undergo surgery. There's a major stressor on your poor body, which has to struggle harder to meet those new demands. Well, guess what? Prolonged stress—whether physical (surgery, illness) or psychological (issues at home or work)—increases your body's metabolic needs. In response to stress, your body wants more vitamin A, C, D, E, and B complex, as well as more minerals, including potassium, magnesium, calcium, selenium, zinc, and chromium. These different needs might well shift your body's definition of friendly and unfriendly foods.

Your dietary needs will always be in flux. Thanks to your diligent work, you now have the tools to understand exactly what your body needs at different times so that you can keep up with your fabulous, ever-changing body.

How to Respond to Seasonal Allergies

So, you've figured out your friendly foods and you're sailing along, losing weight like a rock star. All of a sudden it seems *really* hard to lose weight. And you just happen to have seasonal allergies. Hmmm…Did you know that heightened levels of histamine (and many of the over-the-counter drugs you take for them) can turn you into a weight-gain machine? So what can you do? Slow down your testing. If you were doing well testing two to three times per week, drop down to once a week until things settle down. And if you have a solid food rotation with plenty of friendly foods, then don't test at all until you calm things down a bit.

You've already read about MSM (page 131). For a typical client with seasonal allergies, I recommend starting a six-week course of MSM before allergy symptoms even begin. If you can't manage that, just start when you can and continue for six weeks. You can also add MSM back in any time you notice allergy symptoms start to flare. I'm happy to report that many clients—and me, too!—don't need MSM nearly as often as they thought they would. It seems as though once MSM helps repair your mucosa, the effect of seasonal allergies is greatly mitigated.

Here are your recommended guidelines for MSM.

- If you weigh up to 180 pounds: 3,000 mg/day.
- If you weigh up to 240 pounds: 4,000 mg/day.
- If you weigh more than 300 pounds: 5,000 to 6,000 mg/day.

Every Time You Lose 50 Pounds—Retest!

Boy, do I see this one a *lot*. My patients are so thrilled to find The Metabolism Plan after all those failed diets that they want to just keep on with their friendly foods and avoid everything that didn't work the first time. Ditto with exercise. After all that work, why mess with success?

I'll tell you why. When you lose a large amount of weight, you have created huge beneficial shifts in your body. Your entire biochemistry is different. You've probably corrected some nutritional deficiencies, but your thinner body also just wants and needs different things than the body that was 50 pounds heavier.

So once you have been on The Metabolism Plan for three to six months (the normal time it will take to lose 50 pounds), you should retest. I typically see at least two or three staples that were once your best weight-loss foods suddenly stop working.

Do you need to redo the cleanse when you redo your Plan? The good news is, not unless you want to. You can definitely restart with day 3 and have coffee and wine, but do give chocolate and salt a break on this day.

I know it's scary to test new foods when you may want to keep losing weight, but I am telling you this as a friend. Retest your foods every 50 pounds, and you will *keep* losing weight and achieve your best health.

"What if I Hit a Plateau?"

By now you've probably guessed the four reasons most people hit plateaus:

- They haven't followed the rotation guidelines.
- They haven't retested their foods.

- They aren't hitting their protein counts.
- They aren't exercising in a way that's right for their body.

Just as doing the same workout week after week can cause your progress to come to a screeching halt, so will eating the same foods week after week. So keep remembering to switch it up with both food and exercise.

What you should *not* do if you hit a plateau is cut back on how much you eat or step up the exercise (both can create more stress). Follow the portions given in The Metabolism Plan, and do not increase exercise.

"What if I Hit a Plateau During the 30 Days?"

There's a very good reason why this might happen, and why I don't want you to worry about it. If you're reading this book, you've probably been trying really hard to get to a good weight, for several years or maybe even all of your life. Many people attempt weight loss by beating up their bodies through over-exercise, severe calorie deprivation, or both.

Well, as you now know, stress has taught your body to hold on to weight as a defense mechanism. After all, your body's main goal is to keep you alive. When you program it to think that it will always need a reserve to live off—either because food is scarce or because a lot of exertion is in store—then your body will helpfully try to hold on to your fat for dear life.

So if you have a long history of undereating or have done "deprivation diets," you might well hit a plateau as your body panics and starts preparing for hard times again. I see it in my clients all the time. What I suggest is just go through all 30 days on The Metabolism Plan—but don't cut out foods from the days your weight stays the same, just on the days you gain. By the time you go through all 30 days, your body will start to trust you again and know the famine isn't coming. You can always retest foods later on.

The worst thing you could do would be to start cutting calories, so please keep eating all your portions. Eating less food or ramping up the exercise to an excessive point will only keep this cycle going, dooming you to a lifetime of starvation plus weight gain—the worst of both worlds! Remember, if you are confounded by your data, you can always work with me or one of my staff! (See the Resources section.)

Basically, though, you just need to give your body a chance to realize that the famine is over and the excess stress is gone. When your body trusts that it no longer needs to guard against unhealthy challenges, you'll see the weight loss you've been looking for.

"What if I Start Gaining Weight?"

Okay, confession time. This happens to everyone, even me, for one simple reason: *We haven't retested our friendly foods.*

Once you reach your goal weight, you should stay there—*if* you follow the rules. So if you are one of those rare people who actually does that—if you retest your friendly foods every six months, keep your exercise at the level that your body likes, relieve excessive stress, and are ready to refine your diet as your body changes, you will *not* gain weight.

If, however, you coast along with your friendly foods and forget about retesting them, you *might* start to gain weight, because, sooner or later, one of those friendly foods is going to turn unfriendly.

So if the weight starts to pile back on, if you start to notice that your energy or digestion isn't what it's supposed to be, you can bet that either your food or your exercise has become unfriendly. Use your trusty scale and thermometer, retest your friendly foods and current exercise routine, and figure out what exactly has just stopped working. Now that you have those tools, you never have to feel like you're sliding down a slippery slope. You are in charge. Always.

The last time *I* gained some mysterious weight was about four years ago. For years, my friendliest protein, aside from chicken, had been lamb. Lamb is such a great versatile protein. I could make a large batch of lamb burgers for me and my husband, Bill. I could prepare lamb meatballs for the kids. And all of these dishes could be made up in big batches ahead of time and defrosted at the last minute for a quick and easy dinner. For a busy working mom, lamb's nickname seemed to be Problem Solved.

Well, guess who started to notice they were putting on a little weight? You guessed it: yours truly. And of course I was blaming the fun things, thinking that the problem was too much bread, chips, or cheese.

However, I did notice the one constant seemed to be lamb, so I retested it. And yes, the next day, I gained 0.6 pound.

I couldn't believe it! Not my beloved lamb! We still had three or four lamb dishes waiting for us in the freezer. It was *so* my golden protein—I just had to test it again! So I did—and gained 0.8 pound. My body was speaking loud and clear: *Don't eat this now.*

So lamb and I had to break up. But guess what I *was* able to bring into rotation? Two proteins that hadn't worked in years: wild white-fish and venison. And now, two years later, guess which protein is working again? You got it—lamb!

Over your lifetime, you can always maintain a healthy weight with the foods that you love. You just need to take a break sometimes.

"What if I'm a Vegetarian or Vegan with Low BBT?"

We talked about this in Chapter 2, but it bears repeating: Iron, iodine, and B12 are all essential for a healthy thyroid, and it's hard to get enough of those nutrients on a vegetarian or vegan diet. In your case, supplements might be the way to go, although you've got some food choices as well.

Iodine, which is essential for proper thyroid function, can be found in kelp, which you can add in the form of a seasoning. I like Maine Sea Seasonings, Kelp or Dulse, which comes in shaker form so you can sprinkle a little on your soups or vegetables. It runs only a few dollars and is regularly tested for toxins. Seaweed, alas, though highly nutritious, can also absorb toxins, so if you go this route, make sure you get it only from cleaner waters.

B12 is essential for absorption of iron, as well as for thyroid health and a healthy nervous system. Vegans and vegetarians can have a tendency toward anemia, because it's hard to get sufficient B12 and iron from plant foods alone. So you might want to test nutritional yeast (a stellar source of B12) or supplement with B12 and iron. Many iron supplements cause constipation, but two brands I like that don't are Ferrochel and Floradix. Floradix is in liquid form and is mildly sweet, making it really easy to add to pancake and cookie mixes if your kids are low in iron, too.

The Metabolism Plan for Life

I am so happy you now have your personalized approach to weight loss and health, because nobody, and I mean nobody, knows your body better than you. Not the most brilliant doctor, not your mom—*nobody*. All these years you have been doing "the right thing" or avoiding "the wrong thing," and it just wasn't working. Now you finally have the tools to understand what is happening to your body, every single day. On some level, you always knew exactly what you needed. I'm just helping to shine the light and deciphering a few things.

You've just spent 30 days figuring out your chemistry—and what a great beginning! This will be a lifelong journey, because that's what life is, yes? The only constant is change, and the one thing you can be sure of is that you will always have the opportunity to learn something new tomorrow.

Actually, there is one other thing you can be certain of: As long as you practice the principles of The Metabolism Plan, you can maintain a healthy weight, eating the foods your body loves and enjoying your life. You deserve the best, and I'm so happy to have helped you find your answers.

CHAPTER TWELVE

Recipes

Quick, delicious, and easy-to-prepare recipes: That's how we are going to roll for now! I want you to know that cooking at home is not only awesome for your budget, but the best way to take charge of your weight.

BREAKFASTS

THE METABOLISM PLAN (TMP) SMOOTHIE

Makes 1 serving

½ ripe pear
1 cup blueberries
¼ avocado
¼ cup chia seeds
2 cups Rice Dream or Silk Coconut Milk
Optional: 1 tsp honey or agave
Optional: Vanilla extract and/or cinnamon, to taste

Put all ingredients except milk into a blender. Then add Rice Dream or Silk Coconut Milk. Add honey, vanilla, and/or cinnamon, if desired.
Blend until smooth.

BLUEBERRY COMPOTE

Makes 4 servings

2 cups blueberries
2 cups Silk Coconut Milk or Rice Dream
1 cup chia seeds
1 tbsp agave nectar
1 tsp pure vanilla extract
½ tsp cardamom

Combine all ingredients in a small saucepan and bring to a boil. Reduce heat to simmer and let simmer for 2 to 3 minutes, stirring constantly to prevent the chia from congealing. Let sit for 5 minutes to make a soft compote, or 10 minutes for a firmer one. Serve warm. Refrigerate or freeze unused portions.

APPLE STREUSEL

For our folks who have passed almonds and want a delicious breakfast that tastes like dessert!

Makes 4 servings

Streusel Topping
1½ cups almond flour
⅛ cup brown sugar
1 tsp cinnamon
¼ cup butter at room temperature

Apple Filling
3 apples, cored and chopped into ½-inch pieces
⅛ cup brown sugar
1 tsp cinnamon
½ tsp cardamom
¼ tsp cloves

Preheat oven to 350 °F.

In a small bowl, mix all the ingredients for the streusel topping by hand or using a hand mixer. In a medium bowl, combine all the apple filling ingredients and mix them well. Divide the apple mixture into four 8-ounce baking ramekins and pack them down with ½ inch of streusel topping. Bake for 25 to 30 minutes, until streusel topping is lightly browned. Serve warm or refrigerate.

WARM SPELT FLAKES WITH MANGO-BLUEBERRY SAUCE

Spelt is similar to wheat but easier for many people to digest. Bob's Red Mill makes great spelt flakes to use in this recipe. For even greater savings, you can also find spelt flakes in bulk sections of health food stores.

Makes 3 to 4 servings

4 cups spelt flakes
Optional: 3 cups water for soaking
3 cups water
1 cup chopped mango, fresh or frozen
½ cup blueberries, fresh or frozen
1 tbsp honey or agave nectar
1 tsp fresh lemon juice
½ tsp finely chopped fresh ginger
¼ cup water or coconut milk

Optional: Soak the spelt flakes in water in a large bowl overnight in the refrigerator. Soaking makes them even more digestible.

In a small saucepan combine the 3 cups water, mango, blueberries, honey or agave, lemon juice, and ginger. Bring the fruit mixture to a boil over high heat, then lower the heat and simmer until the fruit is softened and the liquid thickened—about 15 minutes.

Take the spelt (soaked or unsoaked) and put in a small saucepan for 3 to 4 minutes with ¼ cup water or coconut milk. Serve warm, with the warm fruit mixture.

FLAX GRANOLA

Makes 4 servings

1 cup water
2 cups flaxseeds
1 tbsp agave nectar
2 tsp ground cinnamon
1 tsp pure vanilla extract
½ tsp nutmeg
½ cup raisins

If you can soak the flaxseeds overnight, great—they will produce more mucilage and be even better for digestion. But if you're in a rush, you can simply combine water and flaxseeds in a medium bowl, mix well, let sit for 30 minutes, and mix again.

Meanwhile, preheat oven to 275 °F. Add agave, cinnamon, vanilla, nutmeg, and raisins to flaxseeds and mix thoroughly.

Spread the granola in a thin layer on a baking sheet and bake for 50 minutes. Reduce the oven temperature to 225 °F as you remove the baking sheet. Chop up the sheet of granola into clusters, flip them over, and bake an additional 30 to 40 minutes, until all moisture is gone and granola is crispy.

SOUPS

All of The Metabolism Plan soups keep beautifully for the week! You can portion out what you need for the week and freeze whatever is left over.

CARROT GINGER SOUP

Makes 10 to 16 servings

1 tbsp cinnamon
1 tbsp cumin
1 tbsp freshly ground black pepper
1 tsp cloves
1 tsp cardamom
½ tsp turmeric
½ tsp allspice
7 quarts water
⅛ cup extra virgin olive oil
5 lb carrots, chopped
2 large red onions, chopped
3 large zucchini, chopped
8 cloves garlic, peeled
5–6 inches ginger, peeled
Optional: 1 can full-fat coconut milk
Optional: 5 or 6 Vietnamese chili peppers

Put the cinnamon, cumin, pepper, cloves, cardamom, turmeric, and allspice into a dry skillet and sauté over medium heat for 30 seconds, stirring constantly. Put the water into a large soup pot. Add the olive oil, carrots, onions, zucchini, garlic, and ginger to the water, and then add the toasted spices. Bring the water to a boil and let it simmer for 45 minutes, until the carrots are soft. Reserve 4 quarts of the water (called Carrot Essence, page 255) for future soup stocks in freezer. Blend the rest of the soup in batches, according to the size of your blender or food processor. If you like a creamier soup, add the coconut milk. For a spicier soup, add the peppers.

CREAM OF BROCCOLI SOUP

I have cut out all store-bought chicken stock from soup recipes because almost all of them contain MSG or hidden MSG in, for example, yeast extract and chicken flavor. If you have time to make your own, nothing works better than throwing a chicken in a Crock-Pot with 3 to 4 quarts of water, an onion, some sage, ½ teaspoon sea salt, and some white pepper.

Makes 3 to 4 servings

3 tbsp butter

1 large onion, chopped

1 tsp cumin

1 tbsp dried sage

½ tsp dried celery seed

1 quart Carrot Essence (see page 255), or homemade chicken stock, or hot water

2 cups water

1 can full-fat coconut milk

8 cups broccoli, chopped—about 4 heads of broccoli

4 cups zucchini, chopped—about 2 medium zucchini

1 small cayenne pepper or 1 tbsp Sriracha

1 medium avocado, peeled and pit removed

In a medium skillet, melt the butter over medium heat. Add the onion, cumin, sage, and celery seed, and sauté until the onion is tender. To a medium soup pot, add the Carrot Essence or stock, water, coconut milk, broccoli, zucchini, cayenne pepper, avocado, and finally the sautéed onion mixture. Bring the water to a boil and simmer until the vegetables are tender, about 30 minutes. Blend the soup. This recipe freezes well, so it's great to double the recipe to last for two weeks!

LEMON BASIL ESCAROLE SOUP

Makes 4 to 6 servings

1 large white onion, diced fine
½ tsp dried sage
⅛ cup dried basil
¼ cup extra virgin olive oil
½ tsp pink Himalayan salt
1 tsp black pepper
1 quart Carrot Essence (page 255) or homemade chicken stock
1 quart water
1 tsp agave or honey
2 lb carrots, chopped
8 cups zucchini pasta or 8 cups zucchini chopped into small chunks
2 heads escarole, chopped
Juice of 1 lemon or lemon juice to taste

In a large soup pot, sauté the onion, sage, and basil in extra virgin olive oil. Add the Himalayan salt and black pepper, Carrot Essence or stock, water, sweetener, carrots, and zucchini, and let the mixture simmer for 20 minutes. Add chopped escarole and let everything simmer an additional 10 minutes. Top with lemon juice.

CHICKEN KALE SOUP

This should last you one week. Make a double batch and freeze the rest if you want to save time in the kitchen next week!

Makes 4 to 6 servings

1 large white onion, chopped
¼ tsp dried sage
⅛ cup dried basil
½ tsp pink Himalayan salt
1 tsp black pepper
1 quart Carrot Essence (page 255) or homemade chicken stock
2 quarts water

1 tsp agave or honey
2 lb carrots, chopped
8 cups packed kale, chopped
2 chicken thighs with their bones

Add all the ingredients to a soup pot, bring to a boil, and let simmer for 45 minutes. Take out the chicken. Remove the meat from the bone, shred it, and return the meat to the soup. For each 16 ounces of soup, you'll consume about one ounce of chicken. This is low-reactive and will not count as a second animal protein.

CARROT ESSENCE

Makes 8 servings

2 tbsp extra virgin olive oil
2 cups chopped leeks
1 large white onion, finely chopped
3 cloves garlic, minced
1 tbsp dried sage
1 tsp freshly ground black pepper
½ tsp sea salt
4 quarts broth from the Carrot Ginger Soup (page 252)
⅛ cup chopped fresh parsley
1 bay leaf

In a large skillet, put the olive oil, leeks, onion, garlic, sage, pepper, and salt. Sauté everything over medium heat for 2–3 minutes, until the onions become translucent. Meanwhile, to a medium-large soup pot, add the broth from the Carrot Ginger Soup, parsley, and bay leaf, and bring it all to a boil. Then add the sautéed onion mixture. Let everything simmer for 20 minutes. Strain the broth by pouring it through a colander into another pot. Use immediately or freeze into batches.

SIDES

ZUCCHINI PASTA

There are many ways to make zucchini "pasta." You can carve up the zucchini with a mandolin or a vegetable peeler. But my easy, lazy way is to use the Paderno Vegetable Spiralizer, which runs $30 to $40. As an added bonus, the spiralizer is easy for older kids to operate. If you want to eat this type of pasta two or three times in a week, you can: It lasts up to seven days. I love to add any leftovers into my stir-fries toward the end of the week. Of course, you always cook the zucchini before eating it, so it counts as a cooked vegetable. Raw zucchini is very hard on digestion, so cook it until it's tender! In the meal plans, I suggest eating it with kale or basil and Sunflower Pesto (page 262), or with scallions and Manchego, but feel free to get creative with your own friendly pasta sauces!

Makes 4 to 8 servings

4 large zucchini, carved into pasta
1 to 2 tbsp extra virgin olive oil for sautéing

Sauté 3 to 4 cups zucchini pasta in a large hot skillet with 1 to 2 tablespoons extra virgin olive oil for 2 minutes until slightly softened. Immediately remove the pasta from the heat and put it in a large mixing bowl. Toss with toppings of choice.

ROASTED VEGETABLES

These go great with any dinnertime protein, and the leftovers are fabulous on a bed of lettuce plus whatever other vegetable proteins you like for lunch. The roasting tends to bring out the natural sugars in the vegetables, though, so if you have some intestinal yeast or any type of sugar craving, you could find yourself craving these. I suggest limiting them to twice a week.

Makes 4 servings

3 large carrots
1 large zucchini
1 yellow squash
1 head broccoli

1 medium onion
4 to 5 cloves garlic
3 tbsp extra virgin olive oil
Italian herbs, fresh or dried, to taste
Sea salt and freshly ground black pepper to taste

Preheat oven to 375 °F. Chop the vegetables and toss them with the olive oil, herbs, salt, and pepper. If you have time, let the mixture stand for 30 minutes before baking for 30 minutes.

BEET AND CARROT SALAD

I like to make up a big batch of this—it keeps for a week. It's fabulous with lunch and a great option for your "raw vegetable" choice for dinner, since these high-fiber vegetables are terrific for your digestion, your gut bacteria, and your supply of antioxidants. They're also a nice way to enjoy raw vegetables in winter.

Makes 4 to 6 servings

4 large carrots, coarsely grated
1 beet, coarsely grated

Put the carrots and beet in a large bowl separately so colors don't bleed into each other. Dress with your choice from the recipes beginning on page 265, or just go with our old favorites—lemon juice, olive oil, and some dill—which are especially nice with both beets and carrots.

VEGETABLE TIMBALE

I love this timbale as a warm, filling, and satisfying way to eat a wide variety of vegetables, with just a touch of cheesy goodness. You can enjoy it as one of your cooked vegetables at dinner or reheat it for lunch and serve on a bed of lettuce. It keeps for about a week, so you get to cook it once and eat it three times!

Makes 8 servings

2 heads of kale, deveined
1 large zucchini
1 yellow squash

1 yellow onion
2 large carrots
4 to 6 ounces goat cheese
2 ounces grated Manchego
6 shiitake mushrooms

Preheat oven to 400 °F. Use a mandolin or knife to slice the vegetables as thinly as you can. Then layer them like a lasagna in a 9 x 11-inch pan: alternate kale, yellow squash, onions, goat cheese, kale again, then carrots, shiitakes, yellow squash, carrots again, and zucchini. Top with grated Manchego. Cook for 40 minutes or until the top layer of cheese is slightly golden.

SAUCES AND SEASONINGS

INDIAN SPICE RUB

This zingy spice rub will taste delicious on your Day 15 chicken at dinnertime, but you can use it on other proteins and even with your sautéed vegetables or curries once you start creating your own menus. Make up a big batch and put what you don't use in the fridge—it'll keep for six months.

Makes 8 to 14 servings

3 tbsp ground coriander
2 tbsp cumin
1 tbsp turmeric
1 to 2 tbsp brown sugar
¼ tsp sea salt
1 tbsp coarsely ground black pepper
1 tbsp cinnamon
1 tbsp ground ginger
1 tsp cayenne pepper
½ tsp ground cardamom

Combine the coriander, cumin, turmeric, brown sugar, and sea salt. Add the remaining spices, adjusting to taste. Store in your fridge in an airtight container for up to six months.

SPICY ALMOND SATAY

When you start creating your own menus, this is going to be a wonderful addition to your vegetables. As I suggest on page 240, you might make up three days' worth of vegetables and eat them with a different sauce each night—including this one. It's also good on raw vegetables for a snack.

Makes 6 to 8 servings

2 tbsp extra virgin olive oil
1 clove garlic, grated fine
1 tbsp grated fresh ginger
¼ tsp cinnamon
¼ tsp onion powder
¼ tsp cumin
½ cup water
2 tablespoons Sriracha sauce, or to taste
1 tsp brown sugar
¾ cup almond butter

In a medium saucepan, warm up the extra virgin olive oil over medium heat. Add the garlic and spices, keeping the heat low for 2 minutes until garlic is lightly browned. Add water, Sriracha, and brown sugar, then stir for 1 minute. Add in the almond butter, one tablespoon at a time, stirring until thoroughly mixed. Use what you like and store the rest in a closed container in the refrigerator, where it will keep for up to 1 week.

SPICY COCO SAUCE

This is one of your mainstays for serving with kale beginning with your three-day cleanse. But don't stop there—it's delicious on just about any vegetable you can think of, and it's great with rice or other grains. It keeps for about a week, so make up a big batch and use it to jazz up your lunches. Just remember, the combination of coconut milk and animal proteins is a test.

Makes 4 to 6 servings

2 tbsp extra virgin olive oil
1 large onion, chopped
3 to 4 cloves garlic, chopped
1-inch piece fresh ginger, peeled and chopped (about 1 tbsp)
1 tsp cumin
½ tsp coriander
1 tsp cinnamon
½ tsp freshly ground black pepper
½ tsp nutmeg
½ tsp cardamom
¼ tsp allspice
1 tsp brown sugar
1 can coconut milk
2 tbsp Sriracha sauce; for extra spice, add more Sriracha or 1 to 2 hot chilies, chopped
Optional: 1 lemongrass stalk chopped into 1-inch pieces

In a large saucepan, heat the oil. After 30 seconds, sauté the onion and garlic for 1 minute, stirring frequently until they start to brown. Add the ginger, cumin, coriander, cinnamon, black pepper, nutmeg, cardamom, and allspice, and sauté for 1 minute on low heat, until the spices start to smell fragrant. Then add the brown sugar, coconut milk, Sriracha, and lemongrass, if desired, stirring for 30 seconds. Reduce the heat and simmer for 15 to 20 minutes, stirring every 5 minutes. Remove lemongrass before serving.

LOW-REACTIVE TOMATO SAUCE

Makes 3 pints

24 ounces low-sodium bottled tomato sauce
20 ounces Carrot Ginger Soup (page 252)
1 garlic clove, minced
1 tbsp agave or honey
2 tbsp dried basil
1 tbsp oregano
½ tsp rosemary

Combine all ingredients in large saucepan and let simmer for 20 minutes. Let cool and pour into individual containers for freezing.

CARROT GINGER DRESSING

Makes 4–6 servings

2 medium carrots, roughly chopped
1 cup water
3 tbsp peeled, chopped ginger
1 tsp packed light-brown sugar
2 tbsp unseasoned rice vinegar
1 tsp fresh lemon juice
⅛ tsp sea salt
Optional: 1 tsp sesame oil*

Combine the carrots and water in a small saucepan. Bring to a simmer over medium-low heat and cook until tender, about 10 minutes. Reserve ½ cup of the cooking liquid.

Transfer the carrots and reserved cooking liquid to a food processor. Add the ginger, brown sugar, vinegar, lemon juice, salt, and sesame oil if you are using it. Pulse until smooth. This dressing will keep in the refrigerator for five to seven days.

* Sesame oil can be reactive for some people, so you can use this recipe as a test to see if you can tolerate it. Make sure the sesame oil is within its expiration date so it has less chance of being rancid.

SUNFLOWER PESTO

This high-protein sauce is one of my favorite ways to enjoy Zucchini Pasta (page 256)—it's one of my bestsellers with LG Kitchen (see Resources), and we make it in big batches and freeze what we don't immediately need. It's also terrific on any type of steamed or sautéed vegetable, or, in a pinch, with raw vegetables as a protein-packed snack. Store it in your fridge in an airtight container, and it will keep for about two weeks.

Makes 10 to 12 servings

¾ cup raw sunflower seeds

1 cup water

2 cups packed fresh basil leaves, or 1 cup fresh parsley and 1 cup fresh mint

¾ cup extra virgin olive oil

3 cloves garlic, peeled

2 tbsp fresh lemon juice

Optional: Balsamic vinegar for thinning the pesto

Soak the sunflower seeds in water overnight and strain them the next day. Put all ingredients in the bowl of a food processor fitted with an S blade. Purée until smooth. To thin the pesto, add more water or 1 to 2 tablespoons balsamic vinegar.

MANGO SALSA

Mangos are such a special treat, and with this zingy salsa, you can enjoy them all week long. When you start making your own menus, prepare a big batch of veggies and eat them three nights running, each time with a different sauce—including this one! You can also enjoy this salsa on pork or chicken. If you want a cooking break, have your local Chinese restaurant deliver some plain steamed veggies and proteins—no soy sauce, no MSG, no salt—and enjoy them with some mango salsa. If you use paper plates, you won't even have to do the dishes! By the way, if you keep some frozen mango in your freezer, you can make this anytime.

Makes 4 servings

1 whole mango, chopped, or 1 cup frozen mango, thawed
Juice of 1 lime (2 tbsp)
½ small red onion, chopped (¼ cup)
1 small dried red chili pepper, cut into strips
1 tbsp ginger, peeled and grated

Combine all ingredients in small mixing bowl. Serve immediately or refrigerate for up to five days.

SPICY APRICOT GLAZE

This is a fabulous choice for your roast chicken—but, honestly, it's just as good on pork, duck, and fish. I like it so much, I look for excuses to work it into my meal plans! You can make up a batch that lasts in your fridge for two weeks or maybe even longer if you've got an airtight container. Just spread it on your pork or chicken and let the sweet-and-sour tang seep into the meat…*mmmm*!

Makes 8 to 10 servings

½ cup apricot jam
¼ to ½ cup water
1 tbsp Sriracha
2 tsp smoked chipotle powder

Mix ingredients vigorously together. Store leftovers in your fridge in an airtight container.

LEMON DILL SAUCE

This versatile sauce is delicious on vegetables, fish, and chicken. Remember when I told you to make up a big batch of vegetables and serve it over three days with three different sauces? This is one of them! Store in an airtight container in your refrigerator for up to one week.

Makes 4 to 6 servings

2 cloves garlic, peeled
⅛ tsp sea salt
¼ cup fresh dill
1½ tsp freshly ground black pepper
1 lemon, zested and juiced (about 2 to 3 tbsp juice)
½ cup extra virgin olive oil

Add the garlic, salt, dill, pepper, lemon zest, and juice to a food processor. Pulse until coarsely chopped, and then, on a low setting, slowly drizzle in the extra virgin olive oil. Serve immediately.

CRANBERRY CHUTNEY

This sauce is amazing on chicken, lamb, and duck breast. It's also great with cheese for a fancy cheese course with bread or crackers. You should be able to keep it stored in the fridge in an airtight container for up to two weeks. Keep some frozen cranberries in your freezer so you can make this anytime.

Makes 4 servings

1 lb fresh or frozen cranberries
½ cup brown sugar
1 cup water
¼ cup chopped apple
2 tsp cinnamon
2 tsp peeled and grated fresh ginger
½ tsp cardamom
½ tsp allspice
¼ cup almond slivers
½ tsp orange zest

Combine all ingredients except almond slivers and orange zest in a medium saucepan. Bring to a boil, then let simmer for approximately 10 minutes, until cranberries start to pop. Add almonds and orange zest, then stir frequently for 2 minutes to break down the cranberries into a chunky puree.

Salad Dressings

LIME AGAVE VINAIGRETTE

This is the perfect salad dressing for people wishing to avoid vinegar or who have yeast issues. I love it pretty much all the time. There are many organic bottled lemon and lime juices, so feel free to substitute those!

Makes 6 servings

¼ cup lime juice
¼ cup extra virgin olive oil
⅛ cup water
1 tbsp agave nectar
1 crushed garlic clove
Optional: 1 tsp dried dill

Combine all ingredients, stirring thoroughly. Use on top of any salad of your choosing. Will keep refrigerated in an airtight container for up to one week.

BASIL MINT VINAIGRETTE

Hands down, this is my personal favorite. Make up a big batch and enjoy it all week long.

Makes 10 to 12 servings

1 cup extra virgin olive oil
¾ cup balsamic vinegar
½ cup fresh basil
½ cup fresh mint

Put all ingredients in a food processor and blend for 1 minute. Serve immediately or refrigerate for up to one week.

THE METABOLISM PLAN (TMP) CAESAR

The classic Caesar is made with hearts of romaine lettuce, but this tastes amazing on any friendly lettuce. I love it on radicchio with apple!

Makes 8 to 10 servings

¼ cup extra virgin olive oil
2 garlic cloves, peeled and chopped
4 ounces goat cheese
2 tbsp lemon juice
2 tsp fresh black pepper
Optional: 2 tbsp fresh dill or basil

Add all ingredients to a food processor with an S blade and blend until smooth. For a lighter dressing, add water as needed. Use on top of any salad of your choosing. Will keep refrigerated in an airtight container for up to one week.

SNACKS

ALMOND GRABBERS

Makes 10 servings

1 cup almond slivers
¼ cup almond butter
2 tbsp honey
2 tbsp chia seeds
2 tbsp flaxseeds
2 tbsp rice milk
1 tsp pure vanilla extract

Preheat oven to 375 °F.

In a medium bowl, combine all ingredients. Let the mixture sit for 15 minutes to release the mucilage that is so very good for your digestion! Form into 2-inch balls. If the dough isn't sticky enough to do this easily, add a dash more rice milk.

Bake for 12 minutes. If the top is a golden brown, they are done. If not, give them another 3 minutes. Remove from oven and let them cool.

TRAIL MIX

Makes 4 to 8 servings

1 cup sunflower seeds
⅓ cup dried cranberries (sweetened is okay)

Mix the seeds and cranberries together. I suggest dividing them into 4 to 8 servings and storing them in bags so that you can easily take a snack to work or grab one for when you need a snack at home.

SPICY ROASTED PUMPKIN SEEDS

Makes 8 servings

1 cup raw, unsalted pumpkin seeds
2 tbsp extra virgin olive oil
¼ tsp cayenne pepper *or* 1 tsp white pepper for a milder spice
1 tsp onion powder

Preheat oven to 250 °F.

Pour the pumpkin seeds into a medium bowl. Drizzle with the extra virgin olive oil. Add spices, then mix thoroughly. Spread pumpkin seeds onto a large baking sheet in a thin layer. Bake for 15 minutes. Stir the seeds and bake for another 5 minutes. Store in an airtight container in the fridge for 7 to 10 days.

HUMMUS

Makes 6 to 8 servings

2 cups low-sodium canned chickpeas, drained and rinsed
½ cup extra virgin olive oil, plus additional for drizzling
2 tbsp water
2 cloves garlic, peeled
⅛ tsp sea salt
Freshly ground black pepper to taste
2 tsp ground cumin, to taste, plus a sprinkling for garnish
Juice of 1 lemon (about 3 tbsp—or more if desired)
Optional garnish: Chopped fresh parsley

Add all the ingredients to a food processor and blend for 1 minute. Taste and adjust the seasoning (you may want to add more lemon juice). To serve, drizzle with the olive oil and sprinkle with a bit more cumin and some parsley, if desired. Serve immediately or refrigerate for up to five days.

PUMPKIN SEED HUMMUS

Here's a great, quick, easy-to-make dip. I love this one because I am reactive to chickpeas, but love a hummus-style dip!

Makes 6 to 8 servings

3 tbsp extra virgin olive oil
1 cup pumpkin seeds
1 to 2 garlic cloves, chopped
½ tsp cumin
Dash sea salt
1 tsp lemon juice
Optional: Add chipotle powder if you like it spicy

In a medium skillet over medium heat, add the olive oil and then add the pumpkin seeds, garlic, cumin, and sea salt. Stir for 5 to 7 minutes until the seeds are lightly toasted. Add all the ingredients to a food processor. Process until it is a thick, chunky consistency. Serve immediately or store and refrigerate for up to 1 week.

ROASTED ALMONDS

Makes 8 servings

1 cup raw, unsalted almonds
1 tbsp extra virgin olive oil

Preheat oven to 250 °F.

Spread the almonds onto a large baking sheet in a thin layer and drizzle them with the oil. Bake for 10 minutes. Stir and bake for another 5 minutes. Store in an airtight container in the fridge for 7 to 10 days.

APPLE CHIPS

Makes 4 servings

2 medium Granny Smith apples, cored
2 tsp cumin
1 tsp cinnamon
Dash of sea salt

Preheat oven to 200 °F.

Slice the apples on a mandolin or in a food processor. Line a baking sheet with parchment paper and place the apple slices next to each other. Combine the cumin, cinnamon, and salt in a small bowl, and sprinkle the seasoning mixture over the apple slices. Bake the apple chips for 60 minutes, then flip them to the other side and cook for an additional 40 to 50 minutes. You can eat them warm or let them cool. Store in airtight container for up to five days.

ZUCCHINI NOUSH

I came up with this snack because I loved the idea of baba ghanoush, but I react badly to eggplant. You can enjoy this with raw vegetables, low-sodium potato chips, Apple Chips (this page)—or get creative!

Makes 16 to 20 servings

¼ cup extra virgin olive oil
1 large white onion, finely chopped (approximately 2 cups)
¼ cup cumin
1 tbsp pink Himalayan salt
⅛ cup water
5 large zucchini, chopped (approximately 10 cups)
Oil for the baking sheet
Optional: 1 cup sunflower tahini

Add the ¼ cup extra virgin olive oil to a large skillet over medium heat and add onion, cumin, and Himalayan salt. Stir until the spices are thoroughly mixed, then stir in the water. Lower the heat to the lowest setting and let the mixture simmer for 30 minutes, stirring often.

Preheat oven to 325 °F.

Add the zucchini to the skillet with the onion and spices and stir well. Spread the mixture on a well-oiled baking sheet and bake for 40 minutes. Then remove it from the oven and mix it well in a medium mixing bowl. The zucchini will break down to a chunky texture, but if you prefer a creamier snack, you can add 1 cup sunflower tahini. Store it in an airtight container in your fridge, where it will keep for about two weeks.

VEGAN CREAMY KALE DIP

Here's a great snack that you can enjoy with raw vegetables, zucchini pasta, or low-sodium potato chips. You can also use it on cooked vegetables as part of a lunch or side dish.

Makes 12 servings

1 bunch of kale
2 cloves garlic, peeled
1 cup coconut milk
1 cup sunflower tahini

Add the kale, garlic, and coconut milk to a medium sauce pan, and let simmer for 10 minutes. Remove from heat and mix in sunflower tahini. Add all ingredients to a food processor and mix until smooth.

GUACAMOLE

Makes 4 to 6 servings

2 ripe avocados, halved and pitted
½ red onion, minced
Juice of half a lime
⅛ cup water
⅛ tsp sea salt
Fresh black pepper
Optional: ½ tsp chipotle powder, test

Place avocados in a medium bowl. If you aren't serving immediately, reserve the pits. Using a fork, mash the avocados. Add the onion, lime juice, water, salt, pepper, and chipotle powder, if using, continue to blend. Serve immediately or place the pits back into the guacamole to keep it from turning brown.

MAIN COURSES

KALE WITH SPICY COCO SAUCE

Makes 4 servings

2 tbsp extra virgin olive oil
1 large red onion, chopped
4 to 5 large cloves garlic, peeled
1 tbsp grated ginger
1 tsp freshly ground black pepper
1 tsp cumin
½ tsp turmeric
½ tsp coriander
1 head of kale, washed, deveined, and chopped (about 5 to 6 cups)
2 large zucchini, chopped
2 heads broccoli, chopped

1 lb carrots, chopped
4 shiitake mushrooms, diced
1 cup Carrot Essence (page 255) or water
Spicy Coco Sauce (page 260)

Put the oil into an 8-quart soup pot with heat on medium. Add the onion, garlic, ginger, pepper, cumin, turmeric, and coriander, and sauté for 1 minute. Then add the vegetables and stir for 1 or 2 minutes, so that the spice and onion mix is well integrated, and cover the pot. Turn heat to its lowest setting and add the Carrot Essence or water, and let everything simmer for 20 minutes. Finally, add the Spicy Coco Sauce and simmer for an additional 10 minutes, stirring frequently to integrate the flavors.

ROAST CHICKEN

I know that the first 30 days are work, so I am keeping these recipes as simple and flavorful as possible. Whenever you see chicken called for, just roast a chicken or cook up a big batch of chicken thighs, drumsticks, or breasts any way you like. Personally I like to bake them at 375 °F for about 50 to 60 minutes with some basic herbs like basil, white pepper, and a little sea salt. Then you can add your sauces at the end. Voilà—you are a chef! A Crock-Pot version is included below.

Whole Chicken in a Crock-Pot

A busy person's delight, this chicken is so moist and tender you won't believe it!

Makes 8 servings

2 tsp sage
1 tsp dried rosemary
1 tsp tarragon
½ tsp garlic powder
¼ tsp cayenne
½ tsp salt
½ tsp freshly ground black pepper
1 whole cleaned chicken

1 lemon, cut into slices

6 cloves garlic

2 large Spanish onions, cut into large chunks

2 tbsp extra virgin olive oil

Combine the spices in a small bowl. Rub the spice mixture all over the chicken. Place the lemon slices and garlic inside the chicken cavity. Place the onions on the bottom of a Crock-Pot and drizzle oil on top. Place the seasoned chicken on top of onions. Cook for 4 to 5 hours on high.

LAMB BURGERS

Ah, my famous lamb burgers. These are real crowd pleasers, so expect everyone to gobble them up!

Makes 4 servings

1 lb ground lamb

1 zucchini, grated

¼ cup chopped red onion

Optional: Herbs of choice, such as basil, parsley, and rosemary, or use a blend, such as herbes de Provence or a salt-free Italian herb blend

Combine all ingredients in a mixing bowl, form into four patties, and pan-sear in a dry skillet for 6 to 8 minutes, until medium rare.

ROASTED FISH WITH CARROTS, LEEKS, AND LEMON

Serves 3 to 4

1 leek

1 large carrot

4 tbsp extra virgin olive oil

1 whole fish, about 1 pound

⅛ tsp sea salt

1 tsp freshly ground black pepper

1 lemon, cut into very thin slices

¼ cup white wine

Preheat oven to 400 °F.

Slice the leek and carrot into thin strips on the diagonal. The thinner you slice the carrot, the sweeter it will be.

Cover the bottom of a large roasting pan with parchment paper and 2 tablespoons of the oil.

Rub the fish inside and out with 1 tablespoon of the oil and season with the salt and pepper. Add the leek and carrot to the cavity.

Center the fish and place it on half of the lemons. Drizzle it with another tablespoon oil and then top the fish with the rest of the lemons. Pour the wine around the fish and roast for 20 to 25 minutes. You can test the fish by inserting a fork—when the fish has no resistance, it's done. Let rest for 10 minutes, then serve.

PLAN PIZZA

Lavash—an Armenian flatbread that you can get in many Middle Eastern stores—is a great choice for making Plan-friendly pizza, as it often contains no yeast or starter! If you can't find lavash, you can always use pita bread.

Serves 2

Extra virgin olive oil, for brushing
9 × 12-inch lavash
¼ cup Low-Reactive Tomato Sauce (page 261)
⅓ cup grated goat's milk Cheddar
Optional toppings: Chopped fresh basil, rosemary, or oregano

Preheat broiler. Brush pizza pan or baking pan with olive oil and place lavash on pan. Spread tomato sauce on lavash and top with Cheddar. Place under broiler for 4 minutes, or until lightly browned. Top with fresh herbs if you like. Cut into slices and serve warm.

Resources

Essential Support for The Metabolism Plan

The Metabolism Plan Website: Videos, Supplements, Free Document Downloads
http://lyngenet.com/
Facebook
https://www.facebook.com/
TheLynGenetPlan/
Twitter
@Lyngenet
To book with a Certified Metabolism Plan Nutritionist or Personal Trainer, email info@LynGenet.com.

Tools

EatSmart scale
http://www.eatsmartproducts.com/
Omron
https://www.amazon.com/Omron
-HBF-306CN-Fat-Loss-Monitor/
dp/B000FYZMYK
Paderno Spiralizer
http://www.padernousa.
com/4-blade-spiralizer/

Recommended Websites for Meditation

Calm
https://www.calm.com/meditate/
Simple free guided meditations from 2 to 20 minutes
Headspace
https://www.headspace.com
This is a very down-to-earth and user-friendly website. You get a free 10-day trial, then pay a yearly subscription fee.

Websites for Exercise

Fitness Blender
https://fitnessblender.com
http://lyngenet.com

Health and Wellness Professionals

Dr. Nicole Talbot; Family Medicine
http://seguinfamilymedicine.com
(830) 372-5200
Dr. Steven Zodkoy; Chiropractor, Kinesiologist, Nutritionist
http://monmouthadvanced
medicine.com
(732) 308-0099
Dr. Oxana Popescu; Internal Medicine
http://modernmedicalpracticeny
.com
(914) 478-5121

Dr. Martha Seeley; Family
  Medicine
http://www.trhosp.org/seeley
(270) 384-1110
Dr. Jorge Galdamez; Family
  Medicine
http://altamed.org
(888) 499-9303
Dr. Andrew Martorella;
  Endocrinologist
http://manhattan-endocrinology
  .com
(212) 288-2869
Mary Elsea; Chiropractor
http://southboulderchiropractic
  .com
(303) 499-5000
Dr. Lana Selitsky; OB/GYN
http://midtownwomenobgyn.com
(212) 879-4742
Dr. Kathleen Fry; OB/GYN
http://drkathifry.com/
(480) 695-1383
Amanda Sini; Midwife
https://medicine.stonybrook
  medicine.edu/obgyn/
  midwifery/faculty
(631) 444-4000
Dr. Tonia Winchester; Naturopath,
  Kinesiologist; Canada
http://drtoniawinchester.com
(250)585-4455
Dr. Carrie Drzyzga; Functional
  Medicine; Canada
http://functionalmedicineontario
  .com
(613) 824-4224

Acupuncture

Dr. Lap Tsui, LAc.; Aesclepius
  Acupuncture
(212) 677-6682

Janet Bardini, LAc.
http://janetbardini.com
(914) 536-5901
Janet Mixson, LAc.
http://acucamden.com
(912) 882-1200

Books

The Calorie Myth

Wellness

Jonathan Bailor, *New York Times*
  Bestselling Author [Podcast]
http://sanesolution.com/saneshow
David King; Holistic Nutrition
  Podcast
http://http://bit.ly/
  healthywildandfreepodcast
Tournesol Wellness; Holistic
  Therapies
http://tournesolwellness.com
(646) 395-1114
Tejal Asher; Physical Therapy
http://bodymoksha.com
(973) 310-2678

Food Companies

Arrowhead Mills Cereals
http://arrowheadmills.com
Columbia County Bread and
  Granola: Flax Granola and
  Sprouted Breads
https://www.columbia
  countybread.com
LG Kitchen
http://lgkitchennyc.com/
Maine Sea Seasonings
https://www.seaveg.com

References

Akçay, M.N., and Akçay, G. (2003). The presence of the antigliadin antibodies in autoimmune thyroid diseases. *Hepatogastroenterology*, 50, Suppl. 2: cclxxix–cclxxx.

Andersen, H.R., Andersson, A.M., Arnold, S.F., Autrup, H., Barfoed, M., Beresford, N.A., Bjerregaard, P., et al. (1999). Comparison of short-term estrogenicity tests for identification of hormone-disrupting chemicals. *Environmental Health Perspectives*, 107, Suppl. 1: 89–108.

Angeli, A., Minetto, M., Dovio, A., and Paccotti, P. (2004). The over-training syndrome in athletes: A stress-related disorder. *Journal of Endocrinological Investigation*, 27: 603–612.

Balkwill, F., and Mantovani, A. (2001). Inflammation and cancer: Back to Virchow? *Lancet*, 357: 539–545.

Baschetti, R. (1997). Similarity of symptoms in chronic fatigue syndrome and Addison's disease. *European Journal of Clinical Investigation*, 27: 1061–1062.

Baschetti, R. (1999). Fibromyalgia, chronic fatigue syndrome, and Addison disease. *Archives of Internal Medicine*, 159: 2481.

Baylor, L.S., and Hackney, A.C. (2003). Resting thyroid and leptin hormone changes in women following intense, prolonged exercise training. *European Journal of Applied Physiology*, 88: 480–484.

Bolland, M.J., Avenell, A., Baron, J.A., Grey, A., MacLennan, G.S., Gamble, G.D., and Reid, I.R. (2010). Effect of calcium supplements on risk of myocardial infarction and cardiovascular events: Meta-analysis. *BMJ*, 341: c3691.

Bolland, M.J., Grey, A., Gamble, G.D., and Reid, I.R. (2011). Calcium and vitamin D supplements and health outcomes: A reanalysis of the Women's Health Initiative (WHI) limited-access data set. *American Journal of Clinical Nutrition*, 94: 1144–1149.

Campbell, N.R. (1996). How safe are folic acid supplements? *Archives of Internal Medicine*, 156: 1638–1644.

Cellular & Molecular Immunology, 8: 213–225; doi:10.1038/cmi.2010.77; published online: 31 January 2011.

Ciloglu, Figen, et al. (2005). Exercise intensity and its effects on thyroid hormones. *Neuroendocrinology Letters*, 26.6: 830–834.

Collin, P., Salmi, J., Hällström, O., Reunala, T., and Pasternack, A. (1994). Autoimmune thyroid disorders and coeliac disease. *European Journal of Endocrinology*, 130: 137–140.

Coussens, L.M., and Werb, Z. (2002). Inflammation and cancer. *Nature*, 420: 860–867.

Cruz, N.G., Sousa, L.P., Sousa, M.O., Pietrani, N.T., Fernandes, A.P., and Gomes, K.B. (2013). The linkage between inflammation and Type 2 diabetes mellitus. *Diabetes Research and Clinical Practice*, 99: 85–92.

Deligiannis, A., Karamouzis, M., Kouidi, E., Mougios, V., and Kallaras, C. (1993). Plasma TSH, T3, T4 and cortisol responses to swimming at varying water temperatures. *British Journal of Sports Medicine*, 27: 247–250.

Duhig, Thomas J., and McKeag, D. (2009). Thyroid disorders in athletes. *Current sports medicine reports*, 8.1: 16–19.

Duntas, L.H. (2004). Thyroid disease and lipids. *Thyroid*, 12: 287–293.

Fasano, A. (2001) Pathological and therapeutic implications of macromolecule passage through the tight junction. *Tight Junctions* (Boca Raton, FL: CRC Press), 697–722.

Fasano, A., and Shea-Donohue, T. (2005). Mechanisms of disease: The role of intestinal barrier function in the pathogenesis of gastrointestinal autoimmune diseases. *Nature Clinical Practice Gastroenterology and Hepatology*, 2: 416–422.

Fernandez, S.V., Wu, Y.-Z., Russo, I.H., Plass, C., and Russo, J. (2006). The role of DNA methylation in estrogen-induced transformation of human breast epithelial cells. *Proceedings of the American Association for Cancer Research*, 47: 1590.

Gary, K.A., Winokur, A., Douglas, S.D., Kapoor, S., Zaugg, L., and Dinges, D.F. (1996). Total sleep deprivation and the thyroid axis: Effects of sleep and waking activity. *Aviation, Space, and Environmental Medicine*, 67: 513–519.

Groschwitz, K.R., and Hogan, S.P. (2009). Intestinal barrier function: Molecular regulation and disease pathogenesis. *Journal of Allergy and Clinical Immunology*, 124: 3–20.

Hackney, A.C., McMurray, R.G., Judelson, D.A., and Harrell, J.S. (2003). Relationship between caloric intake, body composition, and physical activity to leptin, thyroid hormones, and cortisol in adolescents. *Japanese Journal of Physiology*, 53: 475–479.

Hannuksela, M.L., and Ellahham, S. (2001). Benefits and risks of sauna bathing. *American Journal of Medicine*, 110: 118–126.

Humphries, P., Pretorius, E., and Naude, H. (2008). Direct and indirect cellular effects of aspartame on the brain. *European Journal of Clinical Nutrition*, 62.4: 451–462.

Ijichi, T., Hasegawa, Y., Morishima, T., Kurihara, T., Hamaoka, T., and Goto, K. (2015). Effect of sprint training: Training once daily versus twice every second day. *European Journal of Sport Science*, 15: 143–150.

Laukkanen, T., Khan, H., Zaccardi, F., and Laukkanen, J.A. (2014). Sauna bathing, sudden cardiac death and cause-specific cardiovascular mortality. *Circulation*, 130: A16743.

Messina, M., and Redmond, G. (2006). Effects of soy protein and soybean isoflavones on thyroid function in healthy adults and hypothyroid patients: A review of the relevant literature. *Thyroid*, 16: 249–258.

Middleton Jr., E., Kandaswami, C., and Theoharide, T.C. (2000). The effects of plant flavonoids on mammalian cells: Implications for inflammation, heart disease, and cancer. *Pharmacological Reviews*, 52: 673–751.

Miller, J., and Ulrich, C. (2013). Folic acid and cancer—where are we today? *Lancet*, 381: 974–976.

Muller, A.F., Drexhage, H.A., and Berghout, A. (2001). Postpartum thyroiditis and autoimmune thyroiditis in women of childbearing age: Recent insights and consequences for antenatal and postnatal care. *Endocrine Reviews*, 22: 605–630.

Pirotte, B., Stifkens, F., Kaye, O., Radermacher, L., Putzeys, V., Deflandre, J., and Vijverman, A. (2015). Hypercalcemia and acute renal failure: A case report of vitamin D intoxication. [Article in French.] *Revue Medicale de Liege*, 70: 12–16.

Provenza de Miranda Rohlfs, I.C., Sampaio de Mara, L., Celso de Lima, W., and de Carvalho, T. (2005). Relationship of the overtraining syndrome with stress, fatigue, and serotonin. *Revista Brasileira de Medicina do Esporte*, 11: 333e–337e.

Roberts, H.J. (2004). Aspartame disease: A possible cause for concomitant Graves' disease and pulmonary hypertension. *Texas Heart Institute Journal*, 31.1: 105.

Schedlowski, M., Wiechert, D., Wagner, T.O., and Tewes, U. (1992). Acute psychological stress increases plasma levels of cortisol, prolactin and TSH. *Life Sciences*, 50: 1201–1205.

Schulz, P., Kirschbaum, C., Prubner, J., and Hellhammer, D. (1998). Increased free cortisol secretion after awakening in chronically stressed individuals due to work overload. *Stress Medicine*, 14: 91–97.

Simsch, C., Lormes, W., Petersen, K.G., Baur, S., Liu, Y., Hackney, A.C., Lehmann, M., et al. (2002). Training intensity influences leptin and thyroid hormones in highly trained rowers. *International Journal of Sports Medicine*, 23: 422–427.

Stagnaro-Green, A. (2002). Clinical review 152: Postpartum thyroiditis. *Journal of Clinical Endocrinology and Metabolism*, 87: 4042–4047.

Urhausen, A., Gabriel, H., and Kindermann, W. (1995). Blood hormones as markers of training stress and overtraining. *Sports Medicine*, 20: 251–276.

Wilcox, T.G., and Gray, D.M. (1995). Summary of adverse reactions attributed to aspartame. Department of Health and Human Services memorandum.

Wittert, G.A., Livesey, J.H., Espiner, E.A., and Donald, R.A. (1996). Adaptation of the hypothalamopituitary adrenal axis to chronic exercise stress in humans. *Medicine and Science in Sports and Exercise*, 28: 1015–1019.

Acknowledgments

I am so grateful to my team at Grand Central—Jamie Raab and Sarah Pelz, you are like family! Thank you, Stacey Glick, you're an incredible agent, and it's an honor to work with you.

To my awesome team at The Plan, you have such generous spirits and dedication to making people healthier. Thank you for the work and research you all do!

Index

Note: Italic page numbers refer to illustrations.